eating mindfully

how to end mindless eating &
enjoy a balanced relationship with food

susan albers, psy.d.

New Harbinger Publications, Inc.

Publisher's Note

Distributed in Canada by Raincoast Books.

Copyright © 2003 by Susan Albers
                    New Harbinger Publications, Inc.
                    5674 Shattuck Avenue
                    Oakland, CA 94609

Cover design © 2002 by Lightbourne Images
Edited by Kayla Sussell
Text design by Tracy Marie Carlson

ISBN 1-57224-350-3 Paperback

New Harbinger Publications' Web site address: www.newharbinger.com

08   07   06

10   9   8   7   6

Shortly after I began working as a therapist, I became mindful of the enormous amount of suffering that hunger, weight, and eating issues cause. This book is my attempt to help prevent further suffering and to provide comfort to those already touched by it. For this reason, I dedicate this book to all those who are struggling to overcome mindless eating.

Contents

Part I
Mindfulness of the Mind

Part II
Mindfulness of the Body

Part III
Mindfulness of Feelings

Part IV
Mindfulness of Thoughts

Acknowledgments

A noble person is mindful and thankful for the favors he receives from others

—Buddha

Mindfulness is being dutifully watchful and in touch with all of your actions, thoughts, and feelings. As I write this, I am mindful of how difficult it is for me to express my thanks. I am overwhelmed by the enormity of my gratitude and my inability to adequately describe it in a few sentences. I hope those I mention already know why they are important to me.

I am appreciative of my family. They taught me about compassion for the suffering, particularly the pains of humans and animals. I am most thankful for the opportunities they provided. Thank you to Carmela and Tom Albers, Angie Albers; Linda, Judd, and Paul Serotta. I am also grateful for Jane Lindquist, Jason Greif, Lynne Knobloch-Fedders, Giti Pieper, Brian Kayla, Steven Fink, Eric Lingenfelter, John Bowling and John, Rhonda, and Jim Bowling. I am particularly indebted to Victoria for her friendship and daily encouragement professionally and personally.

To my supervisors and colleagues, I am always mindful of your example and wisdom: Dr. Victoria Gould, Dr. Wendy Settle, Dr. Sandra Rhodes, Dr. Tony Bandele, Dr. Sally Spencer-Thomas, Dr. Sue Steibe-Pasalich, Dr. Savannah McCain, Dr. Trudie Heming, and Dr. Noga Niv. I'd also like to thank New Harbinger Publications, particularly my editors, Kayla Sussell and Catharine Sutker.

Finally, I'd like to acknowledge my clients. I am honored by your trust and thank you for generously sharing your mindful eating strategies with me.

Introduction

How common and effortless it is to eat in an uncontrolled, unaware, *mindless* manner. If you've ever continued to snack when you were full, cut calories despite being hungry, or used guilt to guide your eating, you've experienced mindless eating firsthand. Let's face it. Deciding what to eat is not an easy task. It's so tricky that in the United States eating concerns and weight obsessions have reached epidemic proportions, with serious health consequences for a large part of the population.

What turns an everyday activity like eating into such an overwhelming process? The answer to that question is, of course, a complex one. Throughout the book, we will return to that question with some answers. But the bottom line is this: To make smart, healthy eating choices, your body and mind work together to send you essential clues about what you need and want to eat. These clues give you information about "how much" and "what" to eat. The sensations and emotions that signal when you're full, famished, or just wanting to eat something rich and delicious are a complex combination of bodily and emotional feelings. If you are attentive and responsive to these cues, your eating will be healthy, in control, and well regulated.

Dieting and disliking your body are incredibly detrimental to your emotional, mental, and physical well-being. They inhibit your ability to accurately decode your body's messages and feedback. The dieting mindset is akin to taking a knife and cutting the connection that is your body's only line of communication with your head. The dieting mindset can skew your knowledge of healthy eating so badly that you have no idea of what to eat. Mindless eating is then manifested in two ways. You can either "obsess" or "ignore" internal feedback from both your body and mind, rather than responding thoughtfully to your hunger and to your concern about your health.

In this book, you will learn how mindlessness unknowingly corrupts the way you eat a meal, and how it manifests in a variety of eating problems. You will gain insight into why *mindfulness*, which is, of course, the opposite of mindlessness, can provide you with valuable skills to control the way you eat.

What Is Mindful Eating?

Among many other things, mindful eating includes feeling the saltiness of each potato chip on your fingers as you pick it up, and then the taste of salt when you put the chip on your tongue. It's being aware of and listening to the loud crunch of each bite, and the noise that chewing makes in your head.

When you are eating mindfully, as you eat the chips, you take note of the rough texture against your tongue, and the pressure of your teeth grinding together. You feel your saliva moistening the chips and filling the back of your throat, as the chewed food slides down. Mindful eating is feeling the food in your stomach, and experiencing pleasure from eating it. When you are watchful, you notice how your stomach expands and feels fuller while you are eating. You experience each bite from start to finish. You slow down every aspect of the eating process to be fully aware of its different parts, and to feel connected to it.

This is only one small example of mindful eating. Many others are included throughout the book. The main message to keep in mind while you read the chapters is that the key to changing the way you eat is not to develop discipline over your fork, but to master control of your mind. You can do this by studying and understanding your thinking patterns, emotional moods, and various appetites, instead of allowing your old, habitual thoughts and the desire to eat mindlessly be in control.

The goal of eating mindfully is to know the ins and outs of your hunger. You do this by becoming very well acquainted with every aspect of your body and mind's intricate reactions to food and to the process of eating. The exercises in this book are designed to help you develop tools for knowing how to feed yourself in a controlled manner. They provide strategies for developing a mindful eating stance from which you do not judge yourself or try to change your urge to eat. Instead, you are present and aware of your appetite in-the-moment. Eating with a clear head will help you to prevent yourself from overeating, undereating healthy foods, and consuming unwanted foods.

What Causes Eating Issues?

Mindless eating is not the underlying *cause* of eating problems. Instead, it is the *result* of a variety of other complex body and mind issues. Mindless eating is often the surface level, or a visible sign that another problem needs to be addressed. For example, low-self esteem, body image problems, sluggish metabolism, the absence of control and balance, the social and cultural value of thinness, and overeating caused by emotional problems all contribute to mindless eating and to mindless "dieting."

In cases of severely problematic eating, issues arise from a complex combination of biological factors (sensitivity/temperament, low levels of serotonin); mood disorders (depression, anxiety, obsessive compulsive disorder); psychological factors (perfectionism; other personality characteristics); early traumatic experiences (sexual abuse, divorce, death); family factors (control issues, feeling smothered or abandoned, overt conflict); social factors (relationships, athletic environment, peer group pressure); and media influences (appearance-obsessed culture, airbrushed models).

This book is intended to help you address the variety of factors that contribute to your mindless eating, and to aid you in finding strategies for controlling it. It will also help you heal the underlying factors that cause you to overeat or undereat mindlessly. How do your food issues compare to other people's concerns? When do you know that your eating is an actual "issue"? Do you need to seek additional guidance from a professional? These are pertinent questions. If you've asked yourself any of these questions, you are to be congratulated: You are really in touch with yourself and concerned about your own health and happiness.

You can use this book to assess the intensity of your eating issues. As you read, simply be aware of your reactions. If you diligently digest the contents of the book and find that the exercises really don't work for you, that is useful information. Or you may notice that your behavior seems very similar to the signs discussed. If you don't match the examples, or your actions are much more intense, hold that observation in your awareness. It may be an indication that you could use more personalized professional help. When addressing any kind of problem, people, typically, are at different stages of readiness to adapt their behavior. You may be completely ready to make some changes in your life, or you might need some personalized help with the assistance of a professional just to start the change process.

How to Use This Book

If you think that you engage in mindless eating, or if you describe yourself as a chronic dieter, chaotic eater, or as someone who habitually overeats or undereats, keep on reading, even though you may not see yourself immediately in the examples. You may find it helpful to read through the entire book before attempting any of the exercises. Remember that some exercises may be more appropriate or work better for you than others.

If you believe you are facing more problematic eating patterns, or feel you have a more serious eating disorder, this book can be an excellent resource for you, too. It is not a cheap form of therapy nor is it a substitute for professional counseling. However, it can be a valuable adjunct to ongoing treatment. Bring it to a therapist who works with eating disorders and is highly recommended, and/or to a medical professional, and discuss the exercises. Talk about which exercises work for you and which do not. Working together with a professional, you may be able to counter the factors that are standing in your way.

Often, people believe that they should be able "to do it on their own." Somehow, seeking help signifies failure or is seen as a sign of weakness. I cannot emphasize the contrary view enough. I admire the strength and courage it takes to seek assistance. It means you care about yourself, and it is a sign that you believe there is something inside of you worth nurturing and protecting. Seeking help indicates that you want to live the fullest life possible, and you are willing to take another human being into your confidence to ensure your life will be a happy one. This is a mindful stance, one that is nonjudgmental, open, and receptive to all experience. This is the stance that this book will encourage you to adopt, and, hopefully, it will provide many tools for you to do just that.

The Four Foundations
of Mindfulness

The four foundations of mindfulness are an important aspect of Buddha's teachings. As a young adult, Buddha discovered that mastering mindful eating was essential to his spiritual growth. He had been born into a royal family and, when he was a child, he always ate the most succulent and richest foods that India could offer. He grew plump from all of the feasts he consumed. As a young man, he discovered that all the pleasures he enjoyed at the court could not ensure happiness or protect against sadness. So, when he left his royal life to seek enlightenment and a cure for suffering, he tried fasting. He discovered that fasting or severely restricting his food consumption made him weak, ill, unable to concentrate, and brought him no closer to solving the enigma of suffering. What did the Buddha learn from his days of feasting and famine? He learned that both too much and too little food are detrimental to health and well-being. Control, balance, and understanding the unique needs of your body are essential for a happy, healthy life.

Eating mindfully is not about being more vigilant in your food choices. Nor is it just about diligently watching your calories. That's considered dieting, an approach to eating that is not advocated in this book. Eating mindfully is more complex. It uses the "four foundations of mindfulness" as guides for attending to mind and body signals before, during, and after each meal and snack. Eating mindfully urges you to investigate and become fully aware of your body's appetites, and feelings, and constantly changing mental states during every interaction you have with food. When you eat mindfully, essentially, you bring all of the unconscious, buried forces that dictate how you eat to the surface so your mind can examine them, and you can begin to change them.

What Is Hunger?

Hunger is a biological urge satisfied by the complex interactions between your physiological responses to food, your emotions before, during, and after eating, and your thoughts about your body and self, all in conjunction with your constantly evolving moods and desires and nutrient needs. Having to cope with so many ever-changing variables is one reason you eat so inconsistently.

For example, when sad or bored, you are more likely to eat a lot of pleasurable, filling foods. If you're hungry, but you feel embarrassed and shameful about your body, you may choose to ignore your body's needs, even to starve yourself. Mastering the elements of mindful eating requires you to cultivate a deeper, richer awareness of yourself and your eating habits.

This book is divided into four parts. Each part explores in detail one of the four foundations of mindful eating and provides exercises for adapting and changing that foundation's impact on your eating. When these four foundations remain unconscious, they have an inordinate amount of power and control over the way you feed yourself.

The four foundations are outlined by the Buddha in the *Satipatthana Sutta,* the Great Discourse on the Four Foundations of Mindfulness. The Skill Builders are contemporary ideas tailored to help mindless eaters create a contemplative awareness of the four foundations, as they relate to food. These categories aptly draw attention to aspects of the Self that have been damaged my mindless dieting.

The four foundations of mindful eating are as follows:

- **Mindfulness of Mind:** This includes becoming aware of the many aspects of your mind—your actual thoughts (which may be present as conscious words or images), your memories, and your unconscious (or subconscious) desires and fears. It is essentially the state of your consciousness and your level of attention. At different times, your mind can be distracted, restless, sleepy, clinging to the past, zoned-out, obsessed, scattered, vigilant, or guarded, among many other ways of being. These states are transient, changing from moment to moment, but all the while they create a backdrop for how much you understand, and filtering the way you see the world.

- **Mindfulness of Body:** This includes becoming mindful of as many bodily processes as you can bring into your awareness, i.e., what does hunger feel like? It includes experiencing how food feels in your throat, and the sensation of swallowing it. It includes noting how your body reacts to digesting food, and your stomach's and mind's response when the digestive process is completed. It's acknowledging that your breath, movements, sensations, and postures are powered by food.

- **Mindfulness of Thoughts:** As stated above, thoughts can arise as words or images. They can be like subliminal audiotapes that your mind plays over and over, without your conscious awareness that they are playing. When you are mindful of your thoughts, negative thoughts will lose their power over you.

● **Mindfulness of Feelings:** Just as your thoughts are a part of your mind, so, too, your emotions are a part of your body. The body feels emotions or sensations and transmits the information about what it feels to the brain. Different people feel the same emotion in different ways and in different parts of the body. For example, some people feel sadness as a hole in the belly. They overeat to fill the perceived "hole." To others sadness feels as if their hearts are being squeezed. Some people feel anger as a kind of electrical current coursing through their bodies, while to others anger feels like heat radiating from the chest.

When you practice eating mindfully, you become more aware of how and what you are thinking and how and what you are feeling. Your thoughts and feelings, particularly your feelings about your body, are key players in how and what you eat. The more aware you become of your thoughts and feelings in regard to food issues, the more you will be able to eat mindfully.

Mindfulness of the Mind

It's difficult for me to know when I "should" or "need" to eat. So many things sway my eating habits. At work, I eat snacks my coworkers bring in just because the food is there and I don't want to be rude. At other times, I don't reach for a second helping because I'm wondering if other people are secretly snickering about my weight. I've learned to step back and really ask myself, "Am I hungry at this moment?"

I am attentive and observe what is encouraging or stopping me from eating in that moment.

—Emily

Your state of mind is constantly in flux. The desire to eat is a "transient" state of mind that changes rapidly minute by minute. Mindfulness of your mind teaches you to watch and observe the fluidity of your thoughts, emotions, and most importantly your hunger. Rather than immediately reacting to where your mind is in the present moment, you step back from yourself and evaluate whether you are really hungry or not, and examine the social factors and states of mind that affect your decisions about whether to eat or not, and what to eat.

Mindfulness of the Body

My body clearly tells me when I'm hungry and full. If my stomach is grumbling, it's my body's way of saying I am hungry, and I know I've waited too long to eat. If I overeat, my body complains that it feels sluggish, bloated, and uncomfortable. I listen carefully and respond to my body's requests the first time it asks. I pay attention to what makes my body feel content and energized. Doing that pretty reliably lets me know what I would like to eat.

—Molly

Body mindfulness is attending to every aspect of your inner and outer body. For example, it means paying attention to the way you move, the way you see and touch food, and it means paying attention to vital aspects that you can't see, and often take for granted, like breathing. Body mindfulness encourages appreciating your body's many critical functions, and listening to both your brain and body, which are constantly sending signals to each other, and emitting important physiological feedback about being hungry or full, energy level, feeling states, and nutrient needs. Meditation, breathing exercises, and relaxation are ways to help you understand and translate your body's signals.

Mindfulness of Thoughts

I am most critical of myself inside my head. I might be smiling as I take a second muffin, but my head is saying, "You can't eat that, you're already too fat." When I am mindful of my thoughts, I examine them more closely to see which beliefs are realistic and which ones are just created out of irrational thoughts, judgments, and feeling insecure about how I look.

—Heidi

Like emotions, the desire to eat, food cravings, hunger, and fullness are heavily affected by your thoughts. It is likely that you have a silent dialogue going on in your head that mediates your interactions with food, a voice that says "Eat that" or "Don't eat that" and gives you several reasons why. Thoughts that dictate eating patterns are sometimes clear. At other times they can be subtle, even subconscious. Mindless eaters are particularly affected by their own evaluative, critical, unforgiving, harsh thoughts.

A mindful eater pays attention to and is diligently aware of the deliberations that affect appetite. Raising your awareness of your internal stream of thoughts brings your internal voice that dictates eating behavior into view. Mindfulness of thoughts illuminates how your brain filters incoming information and translates thoughts like, "I am good for not eating that" or "I'm bad" or "I'm fat" into the language of behavior.

Mindfulness of Feelings

I often find myself seeking "comfort" foods that deceptively take away my stress almost immediately. When I am mindful, I opt instead to meditate on what prompted me to seek the comfort in the first place. I acknowledge that a candy bar will make me feel good now, but I also consider how my mood will shift into guilt mode later. I don't allow my feelings to be in complete charge of what I eat.

—Andrew

Food and feelings are tightly interwoven. In the classic chicken-and-egg manner, eating leads to feelings (pleasure, satiation, comfort) and feelings (boredom, stress, pain, loneliness) often instigate or stop eating. Emotions like shame, sadness, feeling overwhelmed or out of control are notorious for skewing healthy eating. For this reason, understanding the relationship between your moods and your appetite is essential for gaining control.

Mindfulness in Everyday Life

Mindfulness is a way of thinking and being in the world that is many centuries old, and has been adopted from Buddhist practices of meditation. The goal of mindfulness is to participate in the present moment in a state of complete awareness of your behaviors, bodily sensations, and experience. It's a "Be here right now" approach to living. A Be-Here-Right-Now stance means you appreciate who you are right now, and stop pining for what you don't have in the present moment. How many times have you wished for or dreamed about having a slimmer body and at the same time forgot to appreciate and live within the body you have?

When you are in a mindful state, you do not judge yourself or try to change who you are. Instead, you simply become more "aware" of yourself and how you interface with the world. A mindful state accepts experience, whether it feels good or bad, as it is in the moment it happens. Why is being mindful so important? Because it is the act of refusing to let the only guaranteed moments of your life slip away.

So often, we shift into an "autopilot" way of being. When you are on autopilot, you react and behave automatically and without conscious thought. The most common examples of behaving in a mindless, autopilot way take place while driving or reading. You suddenly "wake up" and realize that you're driving to work instead of home. You completely missed your exit. Or, you have no memory of what you read in the last three pages. These are serious red flags indicating the presence of mindlessness.

Why is acting in a mindless way a bad thing? Because the behaviors and thoughts that slip out of your awareness are bound to continue. Aspects of yourself that you don't like and are unhealthy will persist without you even knowing it.

If you have mindless eating habits, they are going to remain exactly as they are, unless you become aware of every subtle nuance of the issue. However, when they are in your consciousness, you can think of creative options to change them. Becoming aware is the first step to being in control. Awareness allows you to consider the full range of healthy options that are available to you.

At this very moment, while you are reading, you are being mindful. To read and understand the chapters, you have to shift out of autopilot and attend to the words on the page. Perhaps you are feeling the weight and texture of this book in your hand. Perhaps you are noticing and thinking about your reactions as you read. This is how easy it can be to be mindful.

How Mindfulness Heals

The term "mindfulness" came into use in the sixth century during the Buddha's lifetime. When Buddhism spread across Asia and adapted to the customs and needs of many different countries, the practice of mindfulness remained a core concept. The continued use and popularity of mindfulness practices today attest to their timelessness and to the value of its healing power. Mindfulness is a tool that works to prevent physical illness and disease and promotes rehabilitation and healing, as well as being a treatment for mental health problems.

The Mind-Body Connection

Today, in the West, the mind-body connection has been well documented and extensively researched. It is no secret that healing and treating the mind is as important as nursing the body to health. Mindfulness is currently used in conjunction with medical treatments for illnesses such as cancer, AIDS, anxiety, stress, depression, as well as for chronic pain and sleep problems.

The biological underpinnings are simple. When struggling with an illness, your body's defense system uses all of its resources to target the problem. When you feel pain, either emotional or physical, your natural tendency is to fight against your distress. However, denying and resisting aches and pains raises your stress level and uses energy resources that could be used instead to heal the origin of the illness.

Instead of fighting the pain, mindfulness treatments teach you how to be aware of painful sensations and to manage them one moment at a time. For example, suppose you are suffering from back pain. Instead of being angry or irritated by it, you can observe the source, watch it, and target the painful areas with specific relaxation exercises. You don't ruminate on what your life was like without the pain or how you are going to manage it every single day in the future. You dedicate yourself to coping with the hurting moment by moment.

Healing Your Mind

When you are stressed and emotionally in pain, your body's natural immunity decreases. If you are stressed out about your weight or your out-of-control eating, you may spend more of your time reacting to and dwelling on the painfulness of your problem rather than dealing with it directly. However, resisting all traces of suffering will further limit your ability to overcome stress.

There is wisdom to be learned from suffering. Emotional pain can help you grow by opening your eyes to what you don't like and what you want to be different. Insight is one of the most valuable gifts that mindfulness can offer. When you focus on the here and now, free of distraction, you are empowered to make decisions and free to explore new paths to happiness.

Psychotherapists have begun to realize the benefits and healing power of mindfulness. Mindfulness training is now used to treat depression, personality disorders, drug, alcohol, and sexual addictions, and stress among many other things (Alexander 1997; Hayes et al. 1999; Kabat-Zinn 1990; Linehan 1993; Thich Nhat Hanh 1990; Zindel et al 2001).

A mindful perspective suggests that healing begins by acknowledging and compassionately accepting that something in your life is causing you suffering. Instead of getting angry and irritated about your emotional pain or trying to rid yourself of mental stress, you learn to redirect the influence that pain and stress have over your life. This stance has helped people get through extraordinarily painful conditions, like chronic illnesses, that at first seemed to be overwhelming and beyond control.

There is a notable overlap between mindfulness and cognitive behavior skills. For years, therapists acknowledged cognitive behavioral therapy (interventions that target distorted behavior and thought patterns) as one of the most successful forms of therapy for treating certain eating problems. Recently, therapists have begun to understand the usefulness of mindfulness for developing disciplined, controlled eating patterns (Marcus and McCabe 2002; Wiser and Telch 1999). These researchers and clinicians borrow from Buddhist methods of meditation and mindfulness and skillfully weave them together with their own psychological language and complex treatments.

The approach used in this book is unique, because it outlines a variety of easy-to-understand Buddhist mindfulness techniques that can help you to change and heal yourself. This approach is grounded in the four foundations of mindfulness that were discussed above: mindfulness of mind, mindfulness of body, mindfulness of thoughts, and mindfulness of feelings.

What Kind of Mindless Eater Are You?

This book is for all those who have issues with their weight or who feel unable to control what they eat—that is, all those who eat mindlessly. The following broad categories describe four types of mindless eaters: *the chronic mindless dieter; the mindless undereater; the mindless overeater;* and *the mindless chaotic eater.*

Many people have dealt with some version of generalized mindless eating at various times in their lives. It might have been during childhood, in high school, in the midst of a relationship, or after having a baby. In this book, these people are referred to as the "chronic mindless dieter."

The other types of mindless eaters often face more difficult and hard to solve issues than the chronic mindless dieter does. Overeating, undereating, chronic eating problems, or eating disorders are often accompanied by other psychological problems, which require a high level of consciousness and dedication to change and/or transform.

If the characteristics discussed in the following sections seem familiar to you, it is likely that you are experiencing some form of an eating issue. It should be emphasized, however, that everyone is unique. People may demonstrate similarities in their eating habits, but the specific characteristics and expressions of mindless eating are shaped by your life experiences, culture, and family. Therefore, you need not identify with every characteristic listed. What is more likely is that you will identify with some aspects of each type of mindless eating.

The Chronic Mindless Dieter

After her first baby was born, Alex gained fifteen pounds. She religiously tried each new fad diet that came along, and hunted for new dieting tricks to "get skinny." In the two years after the baby's birth, she bought no new clothes. She wanted to wait until she had shed ten pounds and could fit into a smaller size. She dreamed about having a flat stomach and wearing a sexy, little black dress. She was no stranger to eradicating sugar, fat, and carbohydrates from her diet. Sometimes she even fasted. On one "miracle diet," she ate nothing but cabbage soup and lost a few pounds, but she was unable to maintain the weight loss.

The worst aspect of these diets was that they were completely unrealistic in terms of her lifestyle. When she reduced her carbohydrate intake, she could not bring a quick sandwich for her lunch. Furthermore, she found she couldn't live without pasta and bagels. If she took the fat-free approach, she ate more food and felt less satisfied. She also had difficulty finding food that wasn't filled with sugar to cover the taste of fat-free food.

No diets made sense and she was always "falling off the wagon." When she jumped back on, other people complained that they couldn't invite her to their homes because they never knew what food would be appropriate to serve to her.

Moreover, her conversation was obsessive and boring. She constantly criticized herself when she "cheated" on her diet.

Characteristics of the Chronic Mindless Dieter

Mind

- Vigilant about food intake, scrutinizes food labels
- Categorizes food as "good" or "bad"
- Makes food choices based on hoped-for weight loss, rather than on health
- Eats a lot before starting a diet, and believes the diet will last only for a short period of time

Body

- Engages in yo-yo dieting, leading to constant body weight increase and decrease, which in the long run is very unhealthy
- Is perpetually dieting, and tries out all the new weight-loss gimmicks
- Fasts and cuts back food intake to unhealthy levels
- Doesn't listen to her/his body's desires

Thoughts

- Knows a lot of information about calories, food portions, and diet tricks
- Ignores nutrient needs
- Believes she/he has an "ideal" weight to achieve
- Talks and thinks about food frequently
- Thinks more about the caloric value of food than the experience or joy of eating

Feelings

- Feels fat, disapproves of, and/or is disgusted with her or his own body.

- Experiences mood fluctuations based on eating behavior

- Experiences guilt when she/he "breaks the diet"

- Examines other people's bodies; frequently checks mirrors

- Feels as if she/he "cheated" when she/he eats something that is not part of her/ his diet

- Has difficulty accepting the shape of her or his own body and wishes for someone else's

The Mindless Undereater

Fiona's eating issues began in the seventh grade. As the first girl in her class to reach puberty, she endured extensive teasing about her breasts and rapidly changing body. She wore baggy clothes to avoid others' comments, and to focus attention away from her curvy shape.

As a young adult, Fiona obsessed about eating. She refused to put milk in her coffee if it wasn't fat-free, and she used artificial sweeteners in her cereal to avoid the ten extra calories in real sugar. Eating a handful of chips could send her spiraling into a whirlwind of guilt for the rest of the day. Because she believed that other people evaluated and judged what she ate, she found it particularly painful to eat in front of others. Her friends and relatives constantly nagged her that she looked "too thin." They even acted like "food police," and told her what to eat. Regardless of what everyone said about how "painfully" thin she was, she continued to feel fat and did not enjoy eating.

Characteristics of the Mindless Undereater

Mind

- Restricts food intake or eliminates entire food groups such as all red meats, cheese, or wheat products
- Engages in food rituals or has strict, repetitive, habits for eating. For example, eats only frozen meals, or eating at the same time every day
- Has a strong desire for perfection

Body

- Experiences a significant drop in body weight
- Has a slow metabolism (her/his body burns food very slowly)
- Experiences a variety of physical consequences such as a decrease in heart rate and body temperature, loss of menstrual cycle, etc.
- Is drowsy most of the time; has difficulty concentrating; has low energy

Thoughts

- Preoccupied with appearance
- Feels fat or has a negative body image, in spite of others' statements that she/he is not overweight
- Determines self-worth by weight
- Engages in inflexible and extreme either-or, black-or-white thinking
- Makes constant critical judgments about weight and self

Feelings

- Feels fat, disapproves of, and/or is disgusted with her/his body

- Experiences intense mood fluctuations based on eating behavior

- Experiences guilt when she/he "breaks the diet"

- Examines other people's bodies; frequently checks mirrors

- Feels as if she/he "cheated" when she/he eats something that is not part of her/his diet

- Has difficulty accepting the shape of her or his own body and wishes for someone else's

The Mindless Overeater

Jessie described herself as a "chubby" kid. Other children on the block nicknamed her "Chunk." In her home, food was an extremely complicated issue. Her father, a Holocaust survivor who had experienced the effects of forced starvation, encouraged her to eat as much as possible. Her Italian mother's expression of love was to prepare frequent, large, elaborate meals. In general, the family sat around the dinner table in silence. They ate much more than they talked.

As an adult, Jessie was constantly trying to eat "normally." She described her hunger as "ravenous" and "insatiable." She hoarded cakes, bags of cookies, bagels, and ice cream. She promised herself to eat these foods only for desserts or snacks. But, she could eat an entire cake in one night, without batting an eye, and she often did just that. Eating one cookie was dangerous, because she felt unable to stop until she finished the entire bag. Her eating was "good," unless she had a difficult day at work. If she had a difficult day at work, a late night binge helped her to feel better and not dwell on her feelings of inadequacy. Of course, following the binge, she would feel terribly guilty about all of her overeating.

Characteristics of the Mindless Overeater

Mind

- Knows that her/his eating is out of control
- Believes that she/he is unable to stop eating
- Experiences intense food cravings

Body

- Eats more than "average" during a set period of time
- Eats, chews, and swallows very rapidly; increases or shifts in weight frequently
- Has high blood pressure, fatigue, trouble breathing, high cholesterol level, etc.

Thoughts

- Is cognizant of fullness, but continues eating anyway; avoids scales or discussions of weight or weight loss
- Believes that weight is tied to success and failure
- Engages in supercritical thinking about self and weight

Feelings

- Feels distress over bingeing behavior
- Feels embarrassment that leads to eating small amounts of food when in public, but large amounts when alone
- Feels like a social outcast because of overweight

The Mindless Chaotic Eater

Sam first recognized the severity of his mindless eating patterns when confronted by his roommate, Jim. Jim discovered that Sam stole his food and binged on his stock of candy bars whenever Jim left the apartment. To hide his thefts, Sam would run to the candy store to replace the stolen items. He hoped his roommate wouldn't notice the thefts, until he was caught.

As Sam gobbled up the candy bars, he knew he should stop, but he just kept shoving candy bars into his mouth. After eating an entire box of candy, Sam always felt awful. He ended his binges by making himself throw up or by exercising intensely.

He was afraid to get into a relationship for fear his partner would discover his eating problems. In his last relationship, his partner frequently became angry and tried to make him stop eating so chaotically. Jim ended the relationship because he had lost the ability to know which foods or people were good or bad for him.

Characteristics of the Mindless Chaotic Eater

Mind

- Purchases large amounts of food that are eaten secretively

- Overeats, then purges (vomiting, over-exercising, laxatives, diuretics)

Body

- Experiences extreme fluctuations in weight

- Purges food: pays lengthy visits to the bathroom after eating excessive quantities of food

- Exercises excessively; purchases large quantities of food, diuretic drugs, diet pills

- Has unusual swelling around jaws

- Experiences negative body reactions, such as gastrointestinal problems, bloating, gas, headaches, sore throats

Thoughts

- Thinks about self very critically and negatively
- Experiences self-worth as determined by weight
- Engages in rigid thinking

Feelings

- Experiences intense mood swings
- Fears being or becoming fat
- Doesn't cope well with stress and anxiety

These categories provide a general sense, but not an exhaustive list, of mindless eating types. These are not diagnoses or labels, but ways to help create a simple summary of your eating tendencies. Also, the categories point you toward those aspects of mindfulness that most need your attention.

Mindless dieters often seek strategies to transform their long-term relationship to food and to their body shapes. Undereaters often pay special attention to learning nonjudgmental self-acceptance skills, compassionate thoughts, and the impact of food on their ability to feel joy. Overeaters and chaotic eaters tend to gain valuable insights when they demystify the emotions that are fueling their eating. Overeaters and chaotic eaters often gravitate toward learning control skills and emotional stability.

Part I

Mindfulness of the Mind

The secret of health for both mind and body is not to mourn for the past, not to worry about the future, and not to anticipate troubles, but to live in the present moment wisely and earnestly.

—Buddha

1
Awareness—Awakening Your Mind

The first step to being mindful is to become more "aware" of everything. This is a much more difficult task than you might imagine. It means bringing thoughts and feelings previously out of your awareness into the foreground of your mind. Awareness is often clouded by the many demands of a fast-paced world. Attentiveness to the things you "have to do" takes on a greater priority than what's going on internally. The good news is that developing awareness takes no effort whatsoever. It does not require any action nor do you have to change anything. It merely advises you to reorient where you place your attention or your focus.

Awareness is not only about bringing things into your consciousness but focusing your attention and senses in a special way. Mindfulness is like a mirror. It reflects only what is presently occurring exactly the way it is happening without bias or distortions. It's your *interpretation* of what you see that can distort and twist the image reflected in a mirror. Just notice. Be alert, conscious, and pay attention.

If you are familiar with optical illusions, you're aware that your eyes can deceive you. Your mind works in conjunction with your senses to interpret your surroundings. When information is ambiguous, or there is more than one way to interpret it, you have to choose a way to understand it. At that point, you often fill in missing information based on your past experiences. As a result, you often "see" what you expect to see, rather than what is actually there. Honing in on your sensations and all of the information they can give to you helps you to really examine what you're seeing. If you have enough information, then your mind will not create (or imagine) something that isn't there.

Using your five senses is absolutely essential for mindful awareness. When you first become aware of an object, there is a brief instance of pure awareness just before you identify what it is. That happens when your awareness jumps to alertness via your sense of sight, smell, sound, taste, and touch. You just notice your experience without becoming entangled in it. This is a moment of mindfulness.

One client described an example of awakening her mind. She said that she just turned off the chatter in her head, and turned her awareness toward her eating habits. She changed nothing about the way she ate but simply paid attention to each action and eating sensation. This raised her awareness of her "mindless munching." Previously, she only remembered opening the bag of pretzels and finishing the last few bites. She didn't remember anything in between. Giving her eating behavior the front seat in her mind, rather than the back seat, alerted her to possible ways to transform her eating habits. Paying attention to the juicy smell of a freshly cut apple or the crunchy texture of granola made her snacking both more pleasurable and more controlled.

Skill Builder: Mindful Bites

The following is a classic mindfulness exercise. Mindful eating begins by slowing down and awakening your senses while you are eating. All you need is a comfortable, quiet space and a handful of sunflower seeds. You may also use raisins or a single cookie for this Skill Builder. Place the seeds in your palm. First, become aware of their color and shape. Silently use words to describe to yourself what you see. Compare and contrast each of the seeds. See the shadows, indents, and patterns in their outer skins. Notice their weight and texture against your skin. Do the seeds feel light, heavy, rough, or soft? Do they have regular, consistent shapes and sizes, or are they all different? Next, move some seeds between the tips of your fingers. Feel their edges and shapes and the sensations they produce in your fingers. Contrast this with how you remember them feeling in your palm. Now move the seeds up toward your face and smell them. Observe what comes to mind when you take their odor in to your nostrils. Do they bring to mind a memory or an image? Next, close your eyes and place the seeds in your mouth. Think about what it feels like when you run your tongue around the seeds. As you chew the seeds, do you begin to salivate? Are they crunchy? Observe and describe the taste. Is it sweet, salty, or bitter? What do you hear? Notice the sound of your jaw rotating to chew and the sound of your swallow. Say the word "seed" in your head. Repeat it several times before you swallow. What is the sensation as the seeds slide down your throat?

Skill Builder: Awaken Your Senses

This exercise also helps you access and observe your raw sensations. It can be extremely helpful when you are feeling angry or overwhelmed by what's on your mind, which is the most difficult time to stay with pure sensations and just be aware. This exercise begins with a narrow focus on feelings and expands to reconnect you with the rest of what is going on around you. Here is what to do:

- Notice the ebb and flow of your breathing. Relax. Move around to settle yourself. You are learning how to train your mind to attend only to what is happening in the moment.

- Start with your vision. Say to yourself, "I see . . ." and observe what you see around you. Identify colors, shapes, contrasts in hues and textures. Close your eyes and reproduce what you saw as an image inside your mind's eye.

- Move on to what you hear. Say to yourself, "I hear . . ." and describe the sounds around you.

- Continue on to what you smell, taste, and feel. When you get to your feelings, say to yourself, "I feel. . ." and label your feelings. Remember, you can feel conflicting emotions at the same time. For example, you can feel both happy and sad in the same moment.

- Remember to stay at the level of sensation. Don't analyze or interpret.

This exercise is intended to zap you out of your head and reconnect you with your physical sensations of the environment immediately. Feel the book in your hand, attend to what you smell, acknowledge how the chair you're sitting in feels, and press your feet against the floor. Observe the color of the walls and the details of a picture.

2
Observing What's on Your Mind

After you awaken your awareness, the next task is to step back from your mind and observe it. Your mind is in a permanent state of "go." Thinking, dreaming, scheming, calculating, processing, contemplating are just a few examples of the processes going on in your head. There is a lot of content or "stuff" on your mind, but rarely do you slow down and observe what you do with it.

Observing is like painting a verbal picture of what's going on in your head. But you don't add an extra dab of paint to make it look "better," or erase parts you don't like. You don't paint it the way you think it "should" look. Observing is just seeing it like it is, without judgment or alteration. Watching your mind is also like taking a step aside to look inside it. It's like lifting the lid off the top of a pot. You just take the lid off, peek inside, and see what's stewing in your mind.

Here is a classic example of using observation skills to learn awareness of mindful eating patterns. A woman who was practicing mindful eating exercises told me, "I took ten minutes to decide what to order at my favorite deli. I became aware of my frustration and indecision. I turned on my impartial, watchful attitude to figure out what stood in the way of a simple decision. I observed myself and said, 'I'm negotiating right now. I'm aware that I'm not just thinking about satisfying my hunger. I'm *bargaining* with myself.' I'm saying things like, 'If I don't order the hamburger, I can have a candy bar later. If I have the chicken, then I can order the soup as well.' I didn't judge or criticize myself for doing this. After observing my 'bargaining strategy,' I concluded that the wisest choice would be to stop the negotiating and just choose wisely. Which I did."

It is essential to identify and observe your experience without getting caught up in the content of what you tell yourself. Say you are in a crowded subway, and someone steps on your foot. Whether you interpret it as an accident or an intentional act does not change the sensation or the amount of pain you experience, but your interpretation will affect your mood dramatically. This is how influential your judgment of your experience can be.

Skill Builder: Observe Your Hungry Mind and Your Full Mind

Typically, people are unable to think about anything else besides food when running on an empty stomach. The feeling of an empty stomach wipes out every kind of thought except satisfying the hunger. Hunger distracts your mind from the moment and keeps you from observing and describing your experience.

To do this exercise, conduct a mind experiment. Simply observe what happens inside and outside of yourself when you are hungry as opposed to when you are full. Notice and describe as much detail as possible. Observe thoughts, feelings, and your body.

Observing the Hungry Mind: These are the activities in which the hungry mind engages: planning how to obtain food, craving, desiring, dreaming about a snack, feeling scattered and unable to concentrate, feeling unsatisfied, being distracted by smells, listening intently for coworkers leaving for lunch, watching the clock.

Observing the Comfortably Full Mind: These are the activities in which the comfortably full mind engages: feeling satiated, being able to focus on work, feeling happy, soothed, content, satisfied, warm, at rest, attentive, aware.

3
Moment-to-Moment Eating

Eating a mindful meal means completely focusing your mind on the "process" of eating. You take it moment by moment and focus on the here and now. You begin by looking at the food, noting the different colors and shapes. You really see what is in front of you. Every aspect of the food is noted, from the vivid red of a tomato to the smooth, silky texture of yogurt. You also become aware of the manner in which you reach for the spoon and fork. Food doesn't automatically end up in your mouth. Your entire body is involved in getting it there. You acknowledge grasping and lifting the eating utensils, cutting the meat, and notice how it feels when you open and close your mouth. Moment-to-moment eating means being alert to how you chew, the temperature of the food, the taste, swallowing. It means acknowledging what you hear, such as the food sizzling or steaming, the crunching noise that chewing makes, and the sound produced by slurping through a straw.

Moment-to-moment eating not only makes eating more enjoyable, it is also essential for reducing bingeing and overeating. One woman's constant worry was, "How do I know I'm not going to binge if I give in to one of my cravings?" She had been down that road. When she indulged herself with one chocolate-chip cookie, her drug of choice, she routinely lost control and ate too many, which only strengthened her fear of food. To ease this worry, she used mindful eating skills that slowed down her eating "process." She learned to savor the sweet, rich taste, the mouthwatering smell, and the soft, melting texture of the cookies. When she was really in touch with her body's reactions, she connected with the pleasure.

As she meditated on her food, she realized her desire to eat cookies uncontrollably was really about the lack of richness in her life and wanting to let go and feel pleasure. Her desire to binge would come and go from moment to moment. She learned not to allow the urge to overindulge in food consume her.

Skill Builder:
In-the-Moment Meals

One way to slow down the process of eating is to challenge the way you've always done it. Try eating a meal using a pair of chopsticks instead of your customary utensils. This will force you to take smaller portions, eat more slowly, and look at your food more closely. Touch, describe, and feel your fingers flex and grip the chopsticks. At first, you may have trouble picking up the food. Stay with it. Keep trying. Observe the sensations of picking up the food and placing it in your mouth from moment to moment. Consider each bite to be one snapshot of the total experience.

4
Mindful Meals—
Contemplation of Food

When McDonald's proposed opening a restaurant at the base of an ancient landmark, the Spanish steps in Rome, there was an enormous outcry from the community. Why did they mind so much? Italians are famous for their lengthy, leisurely meals. The presence of a McDonald's threatened this important cultural stance on eating. Eating is an experience. It is not to be rushed, done on the fly, or too fast. American culture often emphasizes the extreme opposite of leisurely dining, inherent in the phrase "fast food."

Slowing down is a foreign concept to many busy individuals. Doing several things simultaneously is considered a more efficient way to do things; for example, talking on the phone while cooking. Doing more than one task at a time is confusing and complex. Often, it increases pressure and inhibits concentration. In the extreme, splitting your attention can be dangerous, as in the case of talking on your cell phone while driving. Eating is an activity performed so automatically that people often read the newspaper, talk, watch TV, and listen to music at the same time they are eating. This severely impairs their ability to be mindful of their eating and to choose foods wisely. The urge to do more than one thing at a time shows how foreign it feels to place your attention on one activity in the here and now.

For example, Alex's eating habits were strongly dictated by convenience. Her food motto was "grab and go." Taking a more mindful approach meant sitting down in one place and connecting with the overall experience. Instead of eating her lunch while answering her e-mail and phone messages, she forced herself to do one thing at a time. When she ate, that was all she did. She focused on the act and process of eating. This dramatically increased her connection to the experience. She really tasted the food, and her brain and stomach were able to register the fact that food had entered her body, and to send her a clear message when she was full. She also made fewer careless mistakes that came about when she divided her attention between working and eating.

Skill Building: Mindful Meals

Start with one mealtime: breakfast, brunch, lunch, or supper. Choose a specific location to eat, such as at your kitchen table or in the lunch room at work. Sit quietly in that area, and don't allow any distractions (i.e., don't get up, place all the food that you intend to eat on the table before starting, don't answer the phone if it rings). To be mindful, you must give your full attention to eating. You act with undivided attention rather than producing "autopilot" behaviors without awareness. Dedicate yourself to experiencing fully whatever you do.

Mindfulness teachers traditionally assign their students to do a walking exercise. This is meant to demonstrate the value of channeling the mind on one activity only. How the students walk, their pace, the movement of their legs, all fade completely out of their awareness when their minds are overrun by other thoughts. The exercise teaches the students not to "think," just to walk and observe. By analogy, if you are eating, just focus on the process of eating and enjoying your meal.

5
Break Mindless Eating Routines

Inflexible eating routines are a common cause of mindless eating. Routines and repetition help to simplify the world. We create categories and lists of what we "like," what we "don't like," and what is "okay" to help us make the sometimes overwhelming decision of what to eat. We like to make these decisions simply and quickly.

When concerned about their weight, people also create other categories, such as "too fattening" or "bad." The downside of routine is that we start to make our choices mindlessly, losing sight of why we eat what we eat. We consume food without diligent thought or true enjoyment. We invent limited menus based on emotional reflexes rather than mindful eating habits.

The most common way my clients divide food is into "safe" or "unsafe" groups. Often, a food is unconsciously assigned to a negative category and stays there unless liberated by the list maker. For example, Amy believed she ate in a healthy manner, until she took a conscious inventory. Her rigid menu consisted mostly of salad and plain bagels. Although she loved a wide variety of foods, she ate these two foods because they are low in fat. Choosing to eat only these two foods answered the emotionally loaded question, "What should I eat?" quickly and thoughtlessly. She feared cheese, meat, and avocados because she read they have high fat contents. She never ate them because of the anxiety they caused. She believed eating them would immediately result in weight gain.

Although her mindless eating routines allowed her to feel guilt-free in the moment, this approach had long-term consequences. She became bored with what she ate, and more importantly, it reduced her intake of crucial protein, vitamins, and minerals. Then, her belief that she "couldn't and shouldn't" eat various foods began to prey on her mind. Ironically, this made her angry. Fighting with herself about the foods she allowed herself to eat drained her energy and robbed her of the joy of eating.

Skill Builder: Create New Eating Habits

1. Make two lists, one of the foods you eat "mindfully," and the other of the foods you eat "mindlessly." Foods eaten "mindlessly" are those you avoid, restrict, define as "bad," those that produce strong emotions of guilt, and/or induce over- or out-of-control eating. Mindful foods may produce emotions, but they are mostly positive or neutral emotions. Mindful foods are eaten willingly, without reservation or fear. If you don't divide foods into these categories consciously, you may have an internal sense of your emotional reactions (carefree eating versus eating that results in guilt, stress, or fear). Getting in touch with the way you react to each of these categories of foods is important. The first step to changing any behavior is to become more aware of it. Bring these categories into your conscious, deliberate thoughts.

2. Next, think about how to take food out of the two categories. Remove the "bad" label from a cookie by giving it a purpose. Is your intention to have a snack? If so, eat the cookie in mindful bites, or use it to satisfy a craving for sweets. Or, give yourself a prescription for a once-a-day dose of a cookie. Start with the foods you eat mindlessly. As you begin to be more comfortable, start to experiment by sampling foods

you've completely cut out of your diet, or foods that you are intensely afraid of or are reluctant to eat. Conquer your fears.

3. Break out of your standard routine. Whether you go to the grocery store and buy the same items week after week, or zoom down the aisles looking for the Specials, do something different. Examine and buy an exotic fruit like a mango, papaya, or an Asian pear. Or, try a loaf of gourmet whole wheat bread. Add a touch of spice and variety to your meals. Walk through the store mindfully examining each item. Be aware of products you've never noticed before. Touch and turn over packages, smell the fruits, examine everything, and buy a new food.

6
Sit Still with Your Pain

Buddhist thought suggests that the desire to escape suffering is one deep emotional root of many issues, particularly mindless eating. Modulating your eating habits can be very taxing on your mood and state of mind. If you eat out of mindless routine habit, it is easy to avoid being present and connected to your eating behavior. Mindful eating requires you to consciously say to yourself, "I choose to change my eating, and I will work through any difficulties," every time you sit down to eat a meal.

One client called on the lyrics of Kenny Rogers' song "The Gambler" to describe how she hid from her fears and never knew when to face them. She felt that identifying exactly when to "hold them," "fold them," "walk away," or "run" wasn't her strongest skill. That is, she had trouble deciding when to run from danger, and when to stand her ground and confront her fears.

If you aren't a "fighter," your natural strategy for surviving in the world may be to flee. Arguments, pain, conflict, difficult projects, and anxiety can be very hard to tolerate. Mindfulness says, "Don't run from life, even from those things that are most painful." Accept experience as it is. Sometimes, the places you go to for escape cause more problems than the place you started from. Don't sprint away from pain before you fully understand what the pain is about. Instead, be mindful by holding on, embracing the pain. Understanding what it is all about will help you to identify solutions for working through it.

Tonya entered therapy to discuss her fear of sexual intimacy. She had developed a suspiciously repetitive dating pattern. When the relationship became physical, she quickly backed away. A mindful approach urged her to examine what she was mindlessly running from. As it turned out, it wasn't sex she feared, but her inability to cope with her self-consciousness about her body. She feared that her body would disgust the men she dated. Weight loss had not increased her self-confidence as she had hoped it would. Tonya was a healthy, desirable weight, but she had not dealt with her emotions and her critical self-judgments. Her relationship problems were "weighing her down" even more than her poor body image.

Skill Builder: Unclutter Your Mind

When you sit down at a cluttered desk, often the first impulse is to clean it. Putting papers into neat piles, eliminating clutter, and creating space foster a sense of relief. Facing your problems rather than avoiding them is like making your messy desk manageable instead of finding another place to sit. Work with what you've got.

Are there feelings, thoughts, or problems you are trying to "escape" or avoid? Have you put something aside hoping it will just get better gradually, without any input from you? Don't push the problem away. Set a few minutes aside to close your eyes and sort through the issue you've been trying to escape. Do this by imagining your mind as your desk. What does your mind look like? What is the messiest area? Do you stuff clutter and bad feelings away in a drawer? Are you obsessed with order? Accept whatever feelings arise. They might be anger, frustration, or pain. Don't think of ways to "fix" it, just acknowledge whatever you feel and sit still with the feelings. Set aside your desire to change the things that trouble you, and just examine what is cluttering up your mind.

7
Live in the Now

Instead of living in the moment, it is extraordinarily easy to become trapped in memories from the past or fantasies about the future. These two mindsets entice you away from being truly present in the moment. The consequence of these mindsets is that we live in a state of "I should have" or "I can't wait until," rather than "I am right here, right now." Stay aware of this truth: the present moment is the only *real* time you ever have.

The past, that stretch of time that includes both your earliest memories and your regret about the words you uttered moments ago, will always be the past. It is unchangeable and the opportunity to alter it is nonexistent. Meditating on the past can be helpful when its purpose is to understand and know yourself better. Reflection on the past, however, is most helpful when it is done with an accepting stance, and the desire to learn from it rather than to change it. Unfortunately, most contemplation of the past is done in a judgmental, "I wish I would have" frame of mind, or involves fantasizing about some incident in the past having a different outcome.

Frequently, food restricters and chronic overeaters have had more than their share of painful past experiences. Not surprisingly, such memories are likely to be ever-present in their minds, consciously or subconsciously. Such memories can draw you away from the present, and tempt you to live in the past, mentally reworking what you "should have done." If this is true for you, it is important to work on treating and healing your pain so that you can enjoy living in your present.

Skill Builder: Living in the Present

In this exercise, you will learn one type of Buddhist meditation for letting go of the past and living in the present.

It is called *Dhyana* meditation. It slows down your mind to prevent you from jumping from one thought to another. The exercise involves a little preparation time. First, think about which events draw your mind away from the present. For example, one woman had trouble letting go of an old relationship. Whenever she felt bad about anything, her former lover came vividly to mind. Then, her memories so overwhelmed everything else going on in her present moment that they kept her stuck in a depressed mood.

In this exercise, choose a thought that often interferes with your ability to live in the moment. It could be a recurring thought about your appearance, or a mistake you made, or an unkindness you experienced. It could be a recurring thought about anything.

Next, imagine a stream flowing down the side of a grassy hill. Picture yourself sitting by the side of the stream watching leaves and twigs float by on the water. You can think about your mind as if it were a flowing stream. Thoughts, like leaves, constantly float by. At the bank of the stream, you can stop the leaves and pick them out of the water, or you can watch them float by you. You can do the same with your thoughts. You can pick one out of your many thoughts and dwell on it, or you can let it float by with all of your other thoughts. Notice when negative thoughts about yourself or your body come into your awareness. Don't react to them. Instead, you can take note of their presence and let them float right by you. If you have a negative thought about your past, picking it up and dwelling on it can trap you in the past and prevent you from living in the moment. If you must reach for that thought, hold it briefly, then visualize tossing it back into the stream. Let it go. Become connected with everything that is happening in your life right now. Acknowledge where you are at this moment.

8
What's on Your Mind?
Not on Your Plate!

One client told a compelling story about her inability to cope with her fear of a small protruding growth inside her stomach. Terrified that it was cancer, she did not go to the doctor. After two years, the benign growth had expanded so much that it weighed close to ten pounds. If she had addressed the problem early on, it could have been removed by a simple, virtually painless, surgical procedure. But letting it grow for as long as she had caused numerous other health problems, nearly insurmountable emotional issues, and social isolation. None of these issues were caused by the growth itself. They were the result of not attending to it. The woman finally had to have extensive, invasive surgery to remove it. Had she continued to ignore it, eventually, it would have killed her.

In a way, we all carry around a type of noncancerous growth. These are the issues that won't kill you, but the longer you avoid dealing with them out of fear, the faster they grow, and the more they weigh you down. Facing some pain in the present can forestall much bigger pain in the future. Addressing a weight issue, or any other problem silently expanding in your body or your psyche, will lighten your mind and heart.

Is food really the issue? Often food is not the true problem, but it is used as a way to visibly manifest other problems. Why use food as a way to express other problems? It is a very visible, easily obtainable, legal, and constantly present substance. Also, unlike drugs and alcohol, food is more socially acceptable as a drug of choice.

Food is something people have to deal with every single day, which makes it one of the most difficult problems to control. Unlike alcohol or drugs, which you can cut out from your life entirely, you cannot stop eating food. Eating mindfully means learning how to fine-tune your food consumption, not how to eliminate it.

Skill Builder: The Issues Beneath Mindless Eating

Visualize a large iceberg in the middle of the Arctic Ocean. Imagine diving under the freezing waters to see where it ends. Mindless eating problems are like icebergs, because it is very hard to see how deep they are and what they hide. The "tip of the iceberg" is the visible aspect of your food consumption: How many times a day you eat, the specific types of foods you consume, and the quantity. But the real question of "why" you eat what you eat is invisible and can be answered only by exploring within yourself.

What is underneath your desire to lose weight? What larger issues make up your weight concerns? A general lack of self-esteem, the irrational belief that "I will be happy if I lose ten pounds," or a desire to exercise control over one aspect of your life? We all know what happens when underlying issues are ignored. Turning away from the issues below the surface can be hazardous and leave you vulnerable to unpredictable, hidden dangers. Becoming aware of the issues that cause you to eat mindlessly will help you to learn how to eat mindfully.

9
The Compassionate Mind

In Buddhist teaching, people are urged to be compassionate, that is, to show respect and love to every single living entity. Since you are a living entity, being compassionate also means having compassion for yourself. Compassion includes having patience, generosity, tolerance, and forgiveness not only for others but also for your own struggles. Compassionate behavior also means letting go of envy, spite, critical attitudes, and the desire for revenge. These are integral aspects of living in a way that does no harm—to others or to yourself. They are fundamental Buddhist principles for living well.

Buddha emphasized that without compassion for yourself, it's impossible to display true kindness and sympathy for others. According to this philosophy, *you yourself, as much as anybody in the entire universe, deserve your love and affection.* No matter who you are, you need and have the right to be treated well. You cannot treat yourself well if you are not gentle and compassionate with yourself about your own issues.

If you've ever talked to anyone about your eating problem, you are probably familiar with how easy it is to lack compassion for yourself. When you've stuffed yourself with food, it's hard to be forgiving and say kind things to yourself. It's difficult to let the overeating go. But self-criticism is the polar opposite of compassion. It often emerges from a lack of understanding. You can probably think of a time when you criticized someone's behavior, and then changed your mind after you heard the whole story. When you develop a sympathetic stance, you can go inside and feel the complexity of your pain.

Skill Builder: Being Mindfully Compassionate

Decide where you need to add more compassion in your life. Start with yourself. Be kind to yourself. When you have a problem, be sympathetic instead of critical. If you eat mindlessly, tell yourself "It's okay," and speak to yourself with compassionate words. People who have eating issues are often much better at feeling compassion for others than for themselves. Think about how forgiving you are of other people. Use this as a guide to what you can say to yourself when you have eaten mindlessly. Buddha instructs us that *one word that brings peace is better than a thousand hollow words.* Remember that compassion helps you to think deeply about what caused the problem. Beating yourself up with criticism only makes you feel worse about yourself, and inhibits your ability to think the issue through. Self-criticism will only prompt another cycle of mindless eating. When you start getting down on yourself, counter the self-criticism with thoughts and statements like these:

- It's okay, next time, it will be easier

- I really do try hard, but I had a really tough day

- It's not my fault. Let's try again

- It's a struggle to be mindful when I feel this way

- I am a great friend and an awesome person

- I understand, I know this is hard

- Everyone makes mistakes

- I am in pain about this, but it will pass

- Being mindful is a process; it takes time

- I want what is best for me

- I love myself—no matter what happens, or what I do

10
Stop Mindless Dieting

In general, "mindless eating" is roughly equivalent to dieting. Dieting is a stellar example of living mindlessly. It urges you to forget about the "now," the difficulty and painfulness of dieting, and to focus on anticipated results in the future. The term dieting implies a *distinct time frame* in which you are sensitively aware of your food choices, but you also anticipate that the necessity to maintain this awareness will end. As you diet, you look forward to the time when you will look better and be able to eat "normally" again.

Dieting forces you to change the quantity and type of food you eat and demands that you neglect the four pillars of mindful eating. The "feeling" pillar is hit particularly hard. Diets squeeze out the joy of eating. If a food tastes or feels good, then it must be "bad." The most mindless of diets are those that encourage eliminating an entire food group, such as the diets that instruct you to completely cut out carbohydrates, dairy, or meat. Such diets are cardboard-like in taste and often lack nutritional balance. Dieting is hard, and when it forbids pleasurable eating, it is bound to fail. Approximately 95 percent of dieters gain back the weight they lost one year later (Zerbe 1995).

The mindlessness of dieting becomes obvious when your body reacts negatively to the absence of well-rounded, nutritional food intake. Anecdotally, dieters report headaches, shakiness, and nausea when they suddenly drop their carbohydrate intake and drastically increase their protein.

Clearly, uncomfortable physical symptoms are the signal that you need a variety of specific foods to help your body work properly. When you experience uncomfortable physical symptoms, something important is out of balance. As a rule, mindless eaters believe dieting discomfort will dissipate or that they will simply get used to living with the discomfort. Overall, dieting destroys delicate connections between the mind and the body.

Eating mindfully does not advocate "eat whatever you want whenever you want," but requires you instead to achieve balance and equilibrium between the four mindful eating pillars—mindfulness of mind, body, thoughts, and feelings. If you eat uncontrollably, your body and mind will revolt. Feeling too full can be as uncomfortable as being too hungry. When you are "stuffed" with food, your body feels sluggish and/or bloated. Your mind may be filled with self-criticism, your emotions are likely to be guilt and self-hatred, and, if you can think at all, your thoughts are likely to circle endlessly around what you just ate, and why you shouldn't have eaten it.

One client described overeating feeling like "an overfilled burrito." She felt that her sides would "spill out," and said it was very difficult to move her cumbersome body around when it was too full. All of this can hopefully be avoided by simply listening and responding to your body's cues while are you eating. When you listen to your body, it tells you how much to eat and when to stop.

Skill Builder: Commit to a Mindful Eating Contract

Adopting a mindful eating approach is a choice and a commitment. It requires a conscious, thoughtful decision. The following contract outlines the basic principles of mindful eating. If you are willing to eat mindfully, and are ready to fully reject dieting, you can begin by learning the ins and outs of the basic philosophy that underlies mindful eating.

Start by reading the contract below. Make a written copy of it. As you are writing it, personalize the language to apply to your own struggles. Sign it to acknowledge that you have made an informed and thoughtful decision. Hang up the contract in your kitchen or dining room, or put it where you will see it every day, so you can read it often. As time goes by, you can change or rewrite it as needed.

Mindful Eating Contract

I agree to eat mindfully. I will eat with diligent thought from this point forward.

I agree to change my attitude toward eating completely, on a full-time basis. I understand that diets don't work.

I agree to think about what I eat moment to moment.

I agree to consider each bite on multiple levels by taking into account the taste, texture, quality, bodily reaction, and sensations I experience when I eat.

I agree to eliminate my diet mentality. I will do this by rejecting dieting advice and books, and by becoming nonjudgmental of myself.

I agree to be nonjudgmental of other people's eating habits, weight, and body shape.

I agree to have compassion for myself.

I agree to be mindful of my speech. I will eliminate terms like "restricting" or "forbidden food" from my vocabulary, and I will start using words like *healthy, natural, organic*, and *energizing*, both in my thoughts and conversations.

I agree that being healthy and living mindfully is my number one goal.

I agree to accept myself and my body as is.

I agree to be aware of the unique eating challenges I face.

I agree to accept how uncomfortable, scary, and wrong it feels to let go of dieting.

Signature: _____

11
Deal with the Blues Mindfully

Nearly everyone is vulnerable to mindless eating because the stress of daily life is one of its most common triggers. For example, Linda came home at 6:00 P.M. every day, stressed out from cold-calling prospective customers, feeling hungry. Even before she took off her coat, she walked directly to the kitchen. She grabbed anything that was within easy reach to cram into her mouth. There were many days when she devoured a steady stream of pretzels and dry cereal until dinner was ready. Then she ate dinner. One day, as she walked into her apartment, she got a phone call. She sat down, took the call, and then sat there thinking about her day. Two hours passed before she realized she was hungry.

Essentially, Linda needed time to relax from her day. She immediately went for food as a way unwinding rather than responding to her hunger (or lack of it). It was obvious that she was more stressed than hungry, judging by the way she grabbed anything. Food can comfort and soothe because it instantly changes what is going on inside and redirects your focus. It is easier to eat mindlessly than to deal directly with the sources of stress.

On the other hand, for another woman, Jane, lack of appetite wasn't a symptom of a single problem but a complex response to the many problems and the intense stress that were overtaking her life. When she was a teenager, Jane had taken care of her alcoholic mother. She had often combed the bars at 3:00 A.M. looking for her mother. As an adult, her life had begun to resemble her mother's misfortunes and mistakes. She got married and then divorced in a very short period of time. She was moody, lacked energy, had trouble sleeping, didn't enjoy her life, and had absolutely no appetite. She ate barely enough to function. It was difficult to figure out whether her mindless undereating was causally related to her problems or was the result of her unhappiness. Fearing that Jane was clinically depressed, her friends urged her to seek counseling.

Sadness, frustration, substance abuse, stress, trauma, sexual and emotional abuse, and anxiety are some of the problems that can make you vulnerable to mindless eating. Therefore, it is important to identify whether you have any mood issues. Sometimes, sharp increases or decreases in hunger are signs of depression or a health problem. A person's eating issues are often the outward signal that the person is experiencing emotional pain. Food often temporarily soothes intense feelings. If this is the case for you, you may need some counseling, because without some professional help, it may be very difficult to change your mindless eating patterns into mindful ones.

Skill Builder: Identifying the Issues

1. Identify life issues that may be affecting either your eating or your mindfulness. If you know what they are, then reading a self-help book may be useful. If you are feeling blue or depressed, try *Feeling Good: The New Mood Therapy* by David Burns (1999). If you have relationship problems, try *Getting the Love You Want* by Harville Hendrix (2001), or if you are anxious, worried, or stressed, try *The Anxiety and Phobia Workbook by Edmund Bourne* (1995). *Full Catastrophe Living: Using the Wisdom of your Body and Mind to Face Stress, Pain and Illness* by Jon Kabat-Zinn (1990) is another excellent book if you are stressed out, or living with chronic pain. To learn more about mindfulness and how to use it in your daily life, try *Eight Mindful Steps to Happiness*

(2001), which is a great book by mindfulness expert Bhante Henepola Gunarantana. Bookstores are lined with hundreds of self-help books. Try to get a recommendation for a book that will be a good match with your needs from a mental health professional.

2. Identify how stress contributes to your mindless eating. Take a stress reduction class.

3. Gather your resources. Consult medical and mental health books, Web sites, and experts.

4. Discuss your problems with your friends. Talk it out. When you listen to others, you may be surprised by the universality of the human experience of pain and suffering.

5. Consult a professional. Counseling can help you identify which issues are complicating and instigating your mindless eating. Contact a professional organization for a referral. For an excellent resource, try www.edreferral.com. Medical and mental health evaluations are critical for under-, over-, and chaotic eating patterns.

12
Mindless Undereating and
the Four Foundations

Mindless undereating is being overly mindful or even obsessed with only one aspect of eating, that of restricting caloric intake to reduce body weight. When you engage in mindless undereating, the desire to be thin supercedes your ability to be mindful of the many other aspects of eating and living (nutrition, health, the experience of eating, the feelings connected to eating). The fear of gaining weight dominates all other factors, and prevents you from eating mindfully or being attuned to the potential damage you may inflict on yourself (missed menstrual cycles, bone loss, electrolyte imbalance, heart problems, etc.).

You may mistakenly think that mindless undereating is actually an example of being extremely mindful, and particularly attentive to your diet. This is incorrect because the mindless undereater is focusing intently on only one aspect of the entire experience of eating. She or he ignores hunger cues and shuns the pleasurable aspects of food.

Mindless undereating can be more dangerous to your health than mindless overeating. The effects of mineral and vitamin loss are often more debilitating over long periods of time. Also, the riskiness of the behavior is masked by the desirability of thinness. No one can see the striking contrast between what mindless eating looks like on the outside and the discomfort and misery the mindless undereater feels on the inside.

Amy's food obsession began during her freshman year of college. All of her social activities centered on food. She was always tempted to "hang out" and snack with friends, rather than do her homework. As a chronic perfectionist, she wanted to be the best. In high school she had been a "star" student, but in college she was surrounded by brilliant peers, which made her feel stupid and inadequate.

During Parents' Weekend, her mother looked at her and asked, "Aren't you looking a little puffy, dear?" Horrified at her mother's question, Amy began restricting her calories to loose the "puffiness" as fast as she could. After two weeks of this, paying attention in class or focusing on any mental task for more than five minutes was nearly impossible. Amy obsessed about her caloric intake and fat grams rather than parties or school work. She stayed in her room and avoided dinner.

Her parents and friends showered her with compliments. They said she looked "fabulous." This only intensified her fear of gaining back the weight she had lost. She taught herself not to be "mindful" of the pains in her stomach, fatigue, obsessions with food, and isolation. She looked good on the outside, but she was miserable on many different dimensions on the inside. Others were blind to her suffering.

Skill Builder: Be Mindful of the Four Pillars

Mindless undereaters and dieters typically focus exclusively on calorie content, fat intake, and tightly controlling their food intake. Being mindful of your eating experience means paying attention to all four pillars (your body, mind, feelings, and your constantly changing mindset (hungry versus not hungry, emotional versus physical hunger, etc.). Start keeping a food diary. Try to write down everything you eat every day for several weeks. If writing down specific amounts significantly increases your anxiety or obsessiveness, just track how eating affects each pillar—your mind, body, thoughts, and feelings. This is also a good exercise for mindless overeaters and chaotic eaters.

The following is an example of how to keep a food diary that takes the four pillars into consideration. Make your meal plan for the entire day a balanced one.

My Mindfulness Food Diary

Example: **Breakfast: Muffin, Orange Juice, Banana**

Mindfulness of Mind: I felt really hungry this morning. I didn't have much to eat last night. I have a lot of demanding things to do today. It was hard to stay focused on eating. I may need to pay more attention to my hunger when I'm really stressed out this way.

Mindfulness of Body: My body felt better after eating this breakfast. I know I should bring a snack to work for 10 o'clock because this won't be enough to carry me through to lunch. At this moment, though, I am not hungry, and I don't feel stuffed. I feel just right.

Mindfulness of Thoughts: I noticed my critical self appeared again and questioned whether I could really "afford" to eat the muffin. Then I had an argument in my head. I reassured myself that it was okay to eat the muffin. I also checked in with my body, which felt fine.

Mindfulness of Feelings: The muffin was great. It was crumbly, sweet, and it made my mouth water. I noticed feeling that I was doing a bad thing because I was taking such pleasure in the muffin. Overall, I felt good about eating it, and I let go of the worry.

Keep this kind of record for an entire day to document every meal and snack you eat. Then, try to keep a food diary for a week—two weeks—a month. You will get a very clear picture of your eating patterns and habits that will be very helpful to you on your journey toward mindful eating all the time.

13:
"Let It Go" Mindfully

We hold on tight to positive, happy experiences, and we avoid negative thoughts and states of mind in the desire to get rid of them quickly. Being mindful is letting experience *just be what it is* without trying to change it. Letting go is accepting things the way they are. You don't have to like your body or enjoy eating mindfully to be able to accept both your body and the practice of eating mindfully.

Often, food problems are highly correlated with control issues. The need for incessant planning is an attempt to achieve a sense of order and control in life. Choosing to "let go" of the things mostly out of your control is one way to handle the situation. A mindful approach relinquishes efforts to dominate people or events that are utterly out of your control, and encourages you to accept change as it happens and take charge of the things that are in your hands. Change is good, natural, and inevitable. The unease that accompanies change often indicates only that life feels "different," but it is not necessarily "worse." Unfamiliarity produces discomfort.

Skill Builder: Small Ways to Let Go

1. The feeling that you have lost control is sometimes interpreted by your mind as "failure." Reconceptualize this feeling as your "Go-With-The-Flow" attitude or "Learning-From-This-Experience."

2. Practice the famous adage, "Know thyself." Be clear on your likes and dislikes. Let go of what you "ought" to want. Tell people you hate riding in the back seat,

and tell your significant other that you would love to get a random call while at work. Let people in.

3. Remind yourself it's okay to have needs. Even fish have needs. They die when they are taken out of the right environment.

4. Practice making decisions, even small ones, such as where you want to go with a group of friends for dinner, or choosing the radio station in the car with conviction, or stating confidently and clearly what you want for a snack.

5. Be more assertive. Sometimes people are afraid to state their opinions for fear of being pushy. Assertiveness means standing up for yourself and your rights. Being aggressive means trampling on the rights of others. There is a big difference.

6. Be clear about your boundaries. Know how much personal space, independence, and control you need.

7. Regain order in other areas of your life. Work out relationship problems. Balance your checkbook.

8. Practice simplicity. Reduce your life to the manageable. Clean out your closet. Sell old furniture, empty out the refrigerator, file old papers and bills. Make your inner and outer environment match. Get rid of the excess, keep the essentials.

Letting go of mindlessly dieting seems unimaginable to chronic dieters. The Buddha taught that cravings and desires keep us stuck and unhappy. To liberate yourself from unhappiness, letting go is necessary. To let go of a dieting mindset, first stop, look at your mindless eating, and examine what you've been chasing after. In the case of weight loss, the desire to shed more and more pounds often comes from wanting to look spectacular, to obtain a romantic partner, to be in control, to achieve perfection, or to raise your self esteem. When you have a specific desire, you begin to cling to it and adopt an "I must have it" attitude: "I want a better body, it's the only way to feel good about myself." But clinging to such a desire causes unhappiness.

Awareness of Stated Desire. *Example:* I want to shed five pounds. I eat mindlessly because my desire is for other people to admire me.

Awareness of Clinging: Because I desire the attention, I'm very aware I haven't lost any weight, which makes me unhappy and angry with myself.

Awareness of Letting Go: If I don't have the desire, I won't be consumed with disappointment. I have control over what I crave and I understand how my relentless desire to be thin is really creating my unhappiness. My body as it is isn't responsible for my feelings. It's my desire to impress other people that creates my dissatisfaction. If I want to be happy, and eat mindfully, I have to choose to let go of the desire to impress, which really fuels my craving for weight loss.

Skill Builder: Letting Go of Dieting

Create a personal, symbolic act to begin the letting go process. One client wrote a letter to herself describing her unrealistic, destructive dieting schemes and her desire to revamp her body. She took the letter, folded it into the shape of a boat, walked to the lake, put it into the water and pushed it, until it sailed away. Later, during the inevitable moments that she was tempted to fall back into mindless dieting, she imagined shoving off her little boat. She remembered her hand pushing it off. Create your own symbolic act to recall in the moments that challenge your ability to let go of your desire to diet.

14
Six Sense Perceptions

Those who practice mindful meditation believe we have six senses, not five. In addition to the obvious five senses (sight, hearing, smell, taste, and touch), mindfulness gurus believe that the most important sensory organ is the mind. Your mind is critical for helping you understand, describe, and interpret what you sense. Your "sixth sense," or mind, is alerted by all your senses tightly woven together, and it interprets what is happening. For this reason, using as many of your senses as is possible helps your mind to grasp the whole of an experience.

Mindlessness is like the state your foot experiences when it falls asleep. It is void of sensation. The function of the growing numbness in your foot is to alert you to the need for movement to restore circulation. The contrast between mindfulness and mindlessness parallels your foot being asleep or awake. At first, you aren't even aware you don't feel anything, but, eventually, the lack of sensation becomes uncomfortable. Similarly, you need all of your senses to be alert to eat sensibly.

Skill Builder: Sensory Meals

Dine at an ethnic restaurant or prepare a recipe from a culture other than your own. This will force you to look beyond the obvious and familiar to see what you might not normally notice. If you cook the meal, choose a recipe with exotic spices. Smell them and savor the experience. Cooking a new recipe helps you to break out of your routine. Remember, change is good.

If you choose to dine out, pick a restaurant that will stretch your senses. (Note: For many people, Chinese food may be too familiar to do this exercise properly.) For example, Ethiopian cooking may encourage you to break out of your typical eating habits. Instead of using utensils, food is scooped up with *injera*, a flat bread shaped rather like a pancake. Using your fingers to carry food to your mouth creates a unique tactile experience unlike any other. Also, in some Asian cultures, it is the norm to loudly slurp soup. Although eating this noisily is taboo in American culture, slurping does add another dimension to experiencing what you are eating.

Using Your Sense of Smell

Paying attention to odors is a wonderful way to improve mindfulness. Your olfactory system is directly connected to your brain. Unlike other sensations, smells travel directly to your brain and are registered immediately, without having to be interpreted. For that reason, odors can awaken your mind quickly and directly.

For example, when you walk into a grade school or a doctor's office, you immediately know where you are by the distinct odor. The smell can be so familiar that you may be flooded with feelings and memories attached to that smell, such as a kid's fear of visiting a doctor's office.

You don't even have to realize that you've perceived a scent for it to have an effect on your mood. For example, a client with an ongoing eating issue became aware of feeling a slight discomfort whenever she talked with one of her friends. She liked her friend, and she couldn't understand why she felt irritable whenever the woman was around. One day, she saw her friend using an atomizer to spray perfume on herself and she asked to smell the atomizer. She was amazed to learn that the perfume was rose-scented.

She made an instant connection. Growing up, she had spent a lot of time alone in her room to avoid her family's fighting. Whenever she escaped to her room, she locked the door and opened the window. There was a magnificent rose-bush directly underneath her bedroom window, but the wonderful scent could not mask the sound of her parents yelling at each other.

Skill Builder: Know Your Nose

When you are out walking, be mindful of smells. Choose a day, and be extremely mindful of the scents around you, the odors of the air, trees, and plants. Take note of the scents when you enter a room, the fragrances people wear, the way clothes that have been wet by rain smell. Pay special attention to your emotional reactions to food smells. Think about how quickly odors can alter your mood and change what is passing through your mind. Find out which scents elevate your mood and which bring you down.

15
Advocate for Mindful Eating

Mindless eating is not just a "girl thing." It is a people problem. However, to some extent, being female significantly increases the likelihood that you will struggle with eating problems. According to some studies, approximately 80 percent of women in America report being unhappy with their appearance (Costin 1999; Smolak, Levine, and Strigel-Moore 1996).

Unfortunately, it is more common for women to be critical of and/or loathe their bodies than to love them. If you could eavesdrop on almost any group of women talking over lunch, you would be likely to hear some reflection on the fat content of their food, or hear them scolding themselves for what they are eating.

Although women are particularly vulnerable, eating problems are rising dramatically among men, too. Approximately 10 percent of those struggling with eating problems are male (Costin 1999). From a clinical perspective, there is almost no difference between the way men and women experience food problems. The underlying issues prompting problematic, mindless eating are nearly identical.

The one way men and women slightly diverge is in how their body image concerns are expressed. Women, who have more fat deposits to facilitate fertility, are more likely to focus on losing that extra fat to become thinner. Men have more lean muscle, and, therefore, tend to focus more on shape and tone. Some researchers suggest it is more difficult for men to acknowledge weight concerns because it was formerly thought to be a white, upper class "women's issue." However, men and women and people of almost all cultures, particularly Westernized societies, are vulnerable to eating issues (Costin 1999).

How important are the messages the media delivers regularly, on the hour, about the need to be thin? It depends. It is difficult not to be affected on some level by the diet ads, the images of air brushed models, and the continual accounts of celebrity weight gains and losses. The not so subtle message that it is essential to be thin to be happy appears to be inescapable. It is aired by almost every TV commercial and featured in all the women's magazines and is creeping its way into men's health magazines. People who struggle with extreme mindless eating are often the most negatively affected by the images of unnaturally thin models and sculptured, muscular men. Mindless eaters focus intently on the overarching message that it is better to be thin than to eat healthy food and live mindfully.

Skill Builder: Reshape Your Eating Culture

Think about your vulnerability to social influences. Are you obsessed with images or ads in fashion magazines? If so, throw them out. Become a critical, educated consumer. When you look at ads, observe your emotional reaction and evaluate how much of it is caused by subliminal sexual messages or the perfect bodies selling the products. It's amazing how superthin models are used to advertise products that have nothing to do with physical fitness. Reduce the power of toxic pro-dieting messages. Compliment ads that use real people. Redirect the energy you use to fuel your self-hatred to being angry at the thinness-obsessed media. Don't accept the message that you can and should change your body. Know that you are not alone. Everyone is confronted by the overvalued desirability of thinness. The social directive, "You Must Be Thin," is a difficult ideology to overcome, but if you learn to eat mindfully, it will have less power over you.

Part II

Mindfulness of the Body

Your body is precious. It is your vehicle for awakening. Treat it with care.... To keep the body in good health is a duty ... otherwise we shall not be able to keep our mind strong and clear.

—Buddha

#16
Meditation: Mindfully Study Your Body's Cues

Meditation is a way of stepping inside yourself. It's like taking a flashlight inside your mind to illuminate your inner world. When meditating, one goal is to calm your body and quiet your mind. Another goal is to connect your mind and body so that they form a unified whole.

Creating wholeness between body and mind is extremely important for those who struggle with food issues. In order to recognize the signals the body sends to the brain, you must allow the communication between your thoughts and your body to flow freely, without obstruction. Sometimes, people value one more than the other, which may lead to an unnecessary split between mind and body.

People rarely "feel" or appreciate their bodies when they are working smoothly. It is common to pay attention to your body only when you feel ill. For example, when you have a cold, you may notice your abilities to taste and smell instantly disappear. As you recover, you attend to what your body feels like when it is working smoothly. Meditation helps people cope with difficulties and suffering by teaching them to focus their thoughts and feelings. It helps them to slow down enough to become aware of their thought processes and their bodies' various behaviors. Most importantly, it helps them learn to relax. According to the psychological principle of "reciprocal inhibition" developed by Joseph Wolpe (1958), it is impossible to be relaxed and tense at the same. Meditation is one way to de-stress and calm your inner world.

Skill Builder: Reconnecting to Your Body

1. Here is an exercise to promote tranquility. It is one type of the many meditation techniques for finding a soothing, calming inner peace and insight. Use it when you are having difficulty making healthy, mindful food choices, or when you are feeling overwhelmed emotionally. First, find a position that allows you to be comfortable but alert. Generally, this means sitting or lying down, but make sure to allow your body to feel naturally at ease.

2. Take several deep breaths and relax. Don't forget to keep breathing deeply.

3. Begin by feeling the places on your body that are in contact with other things. For example, feeling the cushion you're sitting on, your feet resting on the floor, your clothes touching your skin. Be aware of your posture.

4. Direct your attention to your feet. First tense and then relax the muscles of your feet and toes, and become aware of how they feel.

5. Now direct your awareness to move slowly up your legs, past your knees, to your thighs. First tense and then relax the muscles of your legs and thighs.

6. Tense and then relax your butt and your hips.

7. Tense and then relax your stomach muscles and your abdomen.

8. Tense and relax your chest and shoulders.

9. Tense and relax the muscles of your arms.

10. Tense and relax your hands and all of your fingers, down to your fingertips. . .

11. Now, continue with your face. Tense and relax the muscles of your face. Notice the feeling of your tongue inside your mouth, the weight of your eyelids, the heaviness of your neck. Relax your forehead by tensing and letting go. Do the same for your scalp. Move slowly through each region of your entire body, and take note of the places where there is tension. Then release those muscles and relax.

12. If you need assistance, buy a progressive muscle relaxation audiotape to walk you through the process of progressive relaxation.

When you have completed this exercise, and you are completely relaxed, you will be in touch with what your body feels like at rest. This is valuable information. You can use it to help counter the anxious nervousness that may tempt you to engage in mindless eating.

17
Release Body Tension with Mindful Breathing

Mindfulness encourages you to do more of something you already do without any thought or planning whatsoever. Just breathe. Being mindful means attending to the way you inhale and exhale instead of allowing your breathing to slip out of your awareness. When trying to regain control over your mind and body, focusing on your breathing is one of the easiest and most important skills you can practice. You are urged to continue to pay attention to your breathing!

Why is breathing so important? Because deep breathing increases the amount of oxygen your brain and bloodstream receive, which leads to clearer thinking and a stronger connection to your body. Also, when you are aware of inhaling and exhaling, you are engaged with the moment, rather than pushing the moment away. Breathing is the very foundation of living. If you aren't breathing, you've ceased living.

The most obvious sign a person is anxious or feeling uncomfortable is that his or her breathing comes to a sudden halt. "I'm holding my breath" is an expression used on a daily basis. It means "I must stop, wait, and see if it's okay." Overall, paying attention to your breathing helps you to be aware of the moment and in control of how you feel in that moment.

Skill Builder: Take a Breather

This exercise presents a technique for instantly reconnecting your mind to your body. It is easy to do and immediately starts a calming response. Try doing this several times a day. Use this exercise to take a three-minute mini-vacation from your worries.

1. Find a comfortable posture.

2. Bring your awareness to your body. Pay attention to how all the parts of your body feel.

3. Relax, feel your body getting lighter.

4. Devote your attention to your breathing. Stay aware. Observe.

5. Breathe from deep inside your stomach. Put your hands on your stomach and make sure your belly pushes out when you inhale, and pulls in when you exhale. This is called "belly breathing."

6. Imagine that you have a balloon inside your stomach. When you breathe in, imagine the balloon expanding and pushing your stomach out.

7. Note the rhythm of your breathing, its coming and going. Pay attention to the feeling of air moving through your nose.

8. Follow your breathing, don't try to alter it.

9. If you are having difficulty keeping your mind from wandering, count each time you breathe out. One number for each breath. When you reach ten, start over or reverse the count. Feel the difference between counting on the in breaths and the out breaths.

10. Or, don't count and pay attention to the muscles that produce the breath.

11. Pay attention to the way you breathe in different situations, such as when you are walking, running, having sex, relieved, happy, sad, or tired.

12. While you are doing this exercise, in addition to relaxing your body, you are prevented from thinking about anything that might be troubling you during the time you take to do it.

18
Mindfulness of Movement

Be mindful of how your body moves. Eating is the essential element for making your body *go*. Be aware that how well your body functions depends on your food intake. Use your need to move and your energy levels as a gauge for how much food you require to keep your body in action.

Skill Builder: Be Aware of Moving Mindfully

Conduct an observational study of your body and its movements. Choose a week and dedicate it to taking note of how your body interacts with the world. Observe your body as if you were watching it in a film, and from the point of view of the main character.

- You don't have to do anything out of the ordinary, just watch and observe your natural movements.

- Notice the way you eat at meals. Do you take small bites or do you cram your food into your mouth? Do you eat slowly or quickly? Do you eat one food at a time, or do you mix foods together?

- Notice the way you sit. Do you slump or cross your legs one over the other? Do you sit still, or do you shift constantly? Are you relaxed, or does your foot shake? How long can your body sustain sitting in one place?

- Notice the way you move while you talk. Do you use hand gestures? How close do you stand to the person to whom you are speaking? Do you touch others when you talk? Where do you direct your eyes, where do you put your hands, how loud do you talk? What do your nonverbal expressions communicate to others?

- Notice the way your body can be assertive and actively involved in moving around in the world. Focus on and become aware of your very vigorous, dynamic moments, such as running, throwing, yelling, playing sports, making love.

- Notice the way your body transports you. Appreciate the sensations of walking. Focus on how your legs move, their rhythm, pace, and stride.

- Notice the way your body relaxes. Focus on how you stretch and move your arms and legs, and how you twist your neck.

- Notice how you lie down. Do you lie on your stomach, roll over, shift around, or do you stay motionless, not moving at all?

- Notice the way you balance. Does your body have to work to maintain your balance? Be aware of the occasions when you shift your balance and lean against something.

- Notice the internal sensations that accompany your movements. What do your joints and muscles feel? When do they feel sore? When do they feel good?

Consider your body from the micro and macro points of view. Imagine the food you put into your mouth traveling into your stomach, being converted to energy, and used by your nerves to send signals to move your body. Think about how one action, like eating, affects the rest of your body's movements.

19
Mindfully Acknowledge Consequences

Unfortunately, mindless eating has the potential to cause a myriad of health problems. People with eating problems are often aware of the potential physical risks, but they tend to avoid thinking about them. Denial, avoidance, or attributing the detrimental effects of mindless eating to other factors are some of the ways that people cope with the hazards of mindless eating.

It requires approximately 1200 calories a day to prevent your body from going into starvation mode (Sandbeck 1993). In other words, you need this many calories to make your basic bodily functions work: blinking, breathing, sleeping, circulating blood, maintaining a heartbeat. This doesn't include activities like walking, sitting up, thinking, and so forth, which require many more calories. When you lack essential minerals and vitamins, your body struggles to maintain its equilibrium. Mindless undereating and nutritional fluctuations are particularly dangerous because the internal damage is often invisible to the naked eye. Chronic extreme undereating is one of the most lethal mental dosorders. The most extreme result of severe undereating and chronic eating disorders is death (Crow, Praus, and Thuras 1999).

Jessica ignored the health implications of her mindless chaotic eating until she got the results of a routine physical. The doctor expressed concern about her high blood pressure and skyrocketing cholesterol. Jessica was well aware of her labored breathing when she exerted herself physically, but she blamed it on factors other than poor eating habits. After hearing her physician's alarm, it was hard to continue ignoring the warning signs. Jessica finally embraced her heath concerns. She came to understand that, if she avoided dealing with her health immediately, her problems would worsen.

To reduce mindless behavior, focus on the potential physical consequences of your restrictive or excessive eating. Learn to recognize your body's distress signals. Teach yourself to avoid judging yourself harshly, and be mindful of the outcome. Note the difference between judging and predicting the physical consequences. "I ate this whole bowl of chips! How could I be so stupid?" versus "If I binge on all of this junk food, the consequence will be it is very unhealthy for my body, and I will feel bad about doing it." Or "I'm so weak" versus "Eating close to nothing is painful, and hard on my body. When I do this, it increases my risk of hurting my body further."

Skill Builder: Mindfulness of Your Body

Take a step back, observe, and become aware of the sensations within your body. Become mindful of the outcome of mindless eating. Keep track of how many times a month you experience the following physical reactions:

- Weakness
- Chronic tiredness
- Injuries that won't heal
- Cuts or bruises
- Inability to concentrate
- Headaches
- Palpitations, or fluttering, of the heart
- Stomach pain
- Gas

- Sore throat
- Vomiting blood
- Sensitive teeth
- Constipation
- Bloating
- Dehydration
- Dry skin
- Scar on fingers from inducing vomiting
- Aching muscles
- Easily broken bones
- Irregular periods
- Cramps
- Cold
- Lack of energy
- Fainting
- Dizzy
- Bowel movement problems

20
Let Go of Your
Former and/or Future Body

Ruminating on your physique when you were in high school, college, or before you had a baby only increases suffering and mindless eating. It's a waste a time to grieve over the disappearance of your "former" body. Mindfulness embraces change and discourages clinging to the past. Buddha reminded us that "everything changes, nothing remains unchanged."

Dieters are notoriously guilty of fantasizing about their "future" bodies. For example, Elaine began dieting to lose weight for her wedding. She repeatedly imagined herself gliding down the aisle in a slimmer body. Three weeks before her wedding, she panicked because she had not made it to her fantasy body. She spent more time thinking about how she "should" look in her wedding dress, and on her failure to reach her desired weight, than she did about getting married. Her unhappy thoughts about dieting distracted her from her happiness about getting married. Not appreciating and accepting your body in the moment means clinging to the past or fantasizing about the future, both of which effectively erase the present.

Skill Builder: Mindfulness of Mirrors

Let go of former and fantasized images of yourself and be present with who you are in the moment. Work on finding at least one part of yourself you can accept and love now. Look in the mirror and describe yourself aloud. Stay in front of the mirror as long as you can. This can be as short as a few minutes or as long as half an hour. The point is to continue to observe the way you look beyond your typical comfort level. If you feel an urge to turn away, if you feel silly or are uncomfortable, be mindful of that reaction. Observe the complex interaction of the four foundations of mindfulness, your mind's awareness of how you feel and what you think about your body. Unless you are going somewhere special, you often don't slow down enough to really take in your appearance. A bad hair day can draw your attention away from seeing the sparkle in your eyes or the rosy glow of your skin. For this exercise, start with one aspect of your body, such as your hands or neck, and then draw your mindful attention to your entire image. Use all of your observing skills.

One client described her reaction to this exercise. She said, "In the past, looking in the mirror was painful. It was like when you pass your reflection in a store window, and your eyes instantly go to the part of your body you hate to make sure you still hate it. To me, mirrors had become equivalent to shining a spotlight on my thighs. I ignored everything else and focused on the part I disliked the most—my thighs.

"For this mirror exercise, though, I dropped the self-criticism, and stayed with my mindful observations. I described myself in detail, like this: 'I have brown, curly hair that reaches my shoulders, it's light with blonde streaks.' I opened up my awareness to the smooth texture of my skin, and the temperature of the different parts of my body. I felt the roughness of my palms, noticed the shades of color in my lips. I began to use mindless words like 'fat,' and more applicable, specific words like 'curved, straight and oval' to describe my shape. I drew my attention to the scent of my clothes and odor of my perfume. I was tempted to use negative and positive descriptors like 'pretty,' 'ugly,' and 'beautiful' and shortcut words like 'thin' and 'fat.' This exercise helped me to mindfully refocus the spotlight away from my previously dreaded thighs and see the whole me—just as I am, without judgment."

If your mind starts to wander into the past, thinking or imagining what you used to look like, or if it visualizes the future and how you wish you looked, bring yourself back on track. Close your eyes and begin again. See who you are in the present moment.

Skill Builder: Accept Yourself in the Moment

This exercise is about choosing to accept yourself as you are at this very moment, and making a verbal commitment to yourself to accomplish that. It emphasizes "letting go" of your desire to change your body radically. Read these affirmations out loud or just bring them to mind when you are making difficult choices about what to eat or whether to feel guilty about what you have eaten.

Mindful Eating Acceptance Affirmations

Mind

- I *accept* that my eating and weight concerns are creating emotional distress, discomfort, and suffering in my life.

- I choose to *accept* my body and weight as they are at this moment.

- Committing to *accept* myself is a choice only I can make.

Body

- I *accept* that my genetic inheritance strongly influences my body shape and weight.

- I *accept* how important is for me to eat mindfully in order to live a healthy life.

Thoughts

- To *accept* my body and weight does not mean that I am "judging" them to be perfect.

- *Acceptance* comes from within myself. I don't seek it from the outside.

Feelings

- I *accept* that my worth is not reflected by my weight and shape but, rather, my worth is determined by who I am as a whole person.

- *Acceptance* includes rejecting the cultural and social messages I receive about weight.

21
Get Dressed Mindfully

Every day, Julie set her alarm for 5:00 A.M. in order to be at work by 8:00. On average, she squandered two hours each morning getting dressed. This seemingly easy task was a daily nightmare. A snug pair of pants or an outfit that made her "feel fat" sent her spiraling into a bad mood for the rest of the day, and instigated mindless eating. While getting dressed, she felt ashamed, frustrated, irritated, ugly, and just not good enough. Choosing clothes was even more difficult when she had her period. She misperceived normal water retention for weight gain.

People with eating issues often spend hours trying on outfits that "don't make them look fat," and they become obsessed with sizes. Having your mood depend on a number is a very dangerous trap. Sizes are not standardized and they vary between designers. The same woman can wear a size 8 in one pair of pants, and a 12 in another.

Amanda's first step toward recovering from undereating was to throw away her "sick jeans." These were the jeans that fit well when she was starving herself. She had tortured herself by getting them out of the closet and using them to measure how much "fatter" she had become. This instigated mindless eating, and gave rise to negative critical thoughts about herself.

Skill Builder: Dressing for Emotional Success

1. Choose comfortable and stylish clothing. Buy soft, comfy fabrics, like cotton and linen, rather than stiff, starchy materials; choose wool pants rather than spandex or tight jeans, short skirts, or hose. Wear

clothing that feels comfortable. Don't buy anything that is tight on you.

2. Identify one "I look and feel really good in this" outfit. Wear it on the days that you are highly vulnerable to mindless eating or when you feel uncomfortable in your body. Save this outfit for the days you need it.

3. If your clothes feel tight, remember that it may not mean you've gained weight. People experience normal, daily weight fluctuations. Water intake and weather changes can account for slight changes in weight.

4. Investigate different clothing brands. Know which designers make clothes that fit your body shape naturally. Stick with those.

5. Think more about how clothing fits rather than the size. Remember no one can see the label but you.

6. Spend more time accenting other parts of your body such as your hair, makeup, jewelry; buy colors that work well with your skin and eyes.

22
Hunger: Mindfully Listen to Your Body

Sensing whether you are hungry or full is an essential skill for mindful eating. When people either restrict their diets or over-eat, they become accustomed to feeling hungry or too full to the point that they no longer are aware of their true appetites. Or, they teach themselves to ignore hunger cues when they occur. You can do this for only so long before your body floods you with signals you cannot ignore. Mindful hunger means knowing when your body needs to be fed.

For example, Amy had ignored her body's hunger cues for so long, she could no longer determine whether she was full or not. Getting reacquainted with her hunger meant establishing a retraining schedule. First, Amy regulated and reorganized her food intake. She did this with a nutritionist and a doctor to determine what she should eat. Her new menu included vitamin- and mineral-rich foods, snacks she craved, and foods her senses enjoyed, all of which energized her body. When Amy learned to eat mindfully, she recognized how cold, boring, bland, and dry her previous "diet" sandwich had been. Eating it had always left her unsatisfied and hungry. When she added a slice of cheese, lettuce, peppers, tomatoes, and low-fat salad dressing to her basic turkey sandwich, she enjoyed eating it. She began to observe the connections between her feelings, thoughts, and eating.

Skill Builder: Identifying Hunger

When you are about to eat something, ask yourself, "Am I really hungry?" If you do nothing else, meditate on these questions: "Do I need to eat or do I just want to eat?" "Would eating this be an example of mindful or mindless eating?" Wait for at least ten minutes before answering. Listen to your body. Identify the physical cues that tell you when you are hungry. If your stomach is growling, this is a very clear sign of true physical hunger. Sometimes, however, the urge to eat can occur more subtly, with confusing signals such as being unable to concentrate or moodiness. Learn to know how your body tells you what it's really feeling. The following text offers some guidelines for recognizing the difference between mindful physical hunger and mindless emotional hunger.

Mindful Physical Hunger

You are mindfully hungry when your stomach growls; when you eat according to what you have planned to eat for the day; when you eat several meals throughout the day rather than one big meal; when you eat balanced, nutritious meals; and when you eat because you know that you are hungry.

Mindless Emotional Hunger

You are feeding mindless emotional hunger when you eat based on the way you feel emotionally; when you eat even though you are not hungry because the food tastes good; when you eat just because the food is there; when you eat because you are bored, angry, or tired; and when you continue to eat, even though you are full.

23
Mindful Weigh-Ins

Every morning Becky stripped down, tip-toed onto the scale, and anxiously waited for the results. She weighed herself twice just to reconfirm the number. Sometimes, she would weigh herself three times a day. Becky decided to put away her scale for good. She described herself as a "scale addict," and decided to go cold turkey. After a scale-free month, Becky discovered she was much more in tune with her body. With no numbers to rely on, she had to hone in on her internal senses. Knowing how her body felt was essential. Overall, she worried less about eating, calories, and numbers. More importantly, she lowered her anxiety level each morning, and gained more time during the day.

Skill Builder: Scaling Back—
Why Weigh?

Put the scale away. Hide it, trash it, give it away, or tape over the numbers. A mindful approach says that your specific numerical weight is insignificant. Weight focuses only on one aspect of your body, and completely ignores whether you are feeling good, or how your body functions at a particular weight. Learn to think holistically about your body.

If you are unable to separate from your scale or know you will be unable to resist weighing yourself when you find one elsewhere, use mindfulness techniques when weighing yourself. Meditate, breathe, be aware of the process of stepping onto the scale. Follow the feelings and thoughts that arise when you weigh yourself. Don't try to push your feelings away, but embrace them and try to see the influence they have on your mindful or mindless eating. Remember that weight is just the number that says how hard gravity has to work to keep you anchored to the earth. On the moon, you would weigh a lot less. It's just a number. Don't let it keep you down emotionally.

24
Mindful Cravings

After eating a healthy lunch, Jeff had a craving for something sweet. Ice cream had been on his mind all day, but it wasn't part of his "diet," so he searched the kitchen for something else to eat. After a bowl of cereal, several handfuls of chips, and an apple, he finally ate a bowl of chocolate-chunk ice cream. A mindful approach would have given Jeff permission to eat what he really craved. After trying to satisfy his food desire with other foods, he ate the ice cream anyway. The cereal, chips, and apple added many more calories than he would have consumed if he had eaten the ice cream when he became aware of wanting it.

When you crave a particular food, it is likely that your body is sending you an S.O.S. Essentially, a craving is your body sending a message not about what you "want" but about what you may "need." If you crave a hamburger, it is probable that your body is low on protein or fat. If you crave a sweet or a piece of fruit, your body may need the sugar. Cravings are the result of deprivation. Typically, we want what we can't have. If you can have it, you won't insist on having it. Mindfulness is letting go of desire and cravings. The idea is to give your body just enough of what it wants. Sometimes eating a small square of chocolate can satisfy the desire for sugar as well as an entire candy bar. But if you crave an entire candy bar, eat it joyfully and mindfully.

Skill Builder: Mindfulness of Cravings

1. What do you usually crave? If it is chocolate, find a way to satisfy your craving in a mindful way. Keep a

mini-candy bar or a handful of Hershey Kisses to fill that craving. Bring food with you. Having a plan makes you less susceptible to losing control.

2. Remember the adage, "Whatever you resist, persists." Approach cravings consciously.

What do your cravings suggest about your eating? Are your food desires an indication that you are too restrictive with your food? Do your cravings suggest that you are seeking comfort? Discover what your cravings mean, and find healthy ways to satisfy them. Ask yourself the following questions whenever you find yourself craving a particular food:

- How will satisfying my craving affect my body?

- How will satisfying my craving affect my mood?

- How will satisfying my craving affect my thoughts about myself?

#25
Walking or Running
"The Middle Way"

Mindless eaters often struggle with their exercise habits, an issue closely related to eating and body image problems. They frequently wrestle with maintaining a healthy, moderate amount of exercise in their lives. The most common problems result from physical activity that is expressed in two extreme ways. That is, avoiding or obsessing about exercise are both likely to create problems. For example, one woman knew her exercise habits had grown out of control when she was unable to skip her workout even for one day. It was always her highest priority despite other important events in her life. Exercising dominated her life and schedule.

Buddha notes that extreme tendencies occur when you are having difficulty walking "the Middle Way" or finding your balance between two extremes. Mindful living is a pragmatic, flexible approach to finding what works for you. It is not just about ending unhealthy habits but also about finding other positive, physical activities. Identifying what will work for you realistically is essential to exercising mindfully.

Alex, for example, always had good intentions to exercise, but she never seemed to have time, due to her on-the-run lifestyle. When she received her monthly bill from the gym, she hid it under a stack of papers to smother her guilt. She had the same reaction when she examined her body in the mirror. When she saw her protruding stomach and too-tight clothes, she was mortified. Her glances in the mirror lasted only long enough to check that her clothing matched. She posted a photo of herself as a teenager on her refrigerator to motivate herself to lose some weight, but the picture only increased her awful feelings about her body. She subconsciously trained her eyes not to see the image of her former self.

When she was honest with herself, she realized that she was too overwhelmed with work to go to the gym every day. She stopped avoiding the bills and faced her feelings. Then she gave up feeling guilty and terminated her membership. Gradually, she began doing physical activities that were more compatible with her lifestyle. For example, she had been taking a streetcar and a bus to get to work. Instead, she began walking to the bus instead of riding on the streetcar. That way she got a good walk twice a day. While walking, she focused on her body's movements and all the sensations of walking.

Skill Builder: Acknowledge Exercise Avoidance

1. Listen to your body. Identify what is realistic for your life. Make a commitment to a "do-able" type and amount of exercise.

2. Start *small* and work your way up. Focus on achievable exercise goals. Once you reach your first goal, bump it up only slightly. "Slightly" is the key word. Increase your exercise only after you've fully mastered that first goal. The most common mistake is to expect too much at once. Failing at an unrealistic, unachievable goal will cripple your motivation. Setting and reaching goals is the best way to keep exercising and gain a sense of accomplishment.

3. What feelings arise when you think about exercise? Use this question to identify what you need to change about your exercise routines. If you are bored, add some excitement by taking a salsa class or buying a

workout CD. If aerobics make you too tired, do low impact exercise.

4. If you can't commit to an exercise schedule by yourself, work out with a friend. If it is painful, slow down, and do something more suitable to your pace.

5. Make small but daily changes to get yourself to move more often. For example, park in the back of the parking lot, which will force you to walk more. Take the stairs instead of the elevator.

When to Say "When"

Not all exercise is healthy. When done excessively, it can turn a healthy behavior into a harmful one. For example, exercise played an important role in John's life. He exercised religiously three hours a day after bouts of mindless overeating. It served as a stress reliever and reduced his anxiety about consuming so many excess calories. However, when he became sensitively aware and mindful of his body, his sore muscles and aching joints were a clear message to stop overexercising. He learned to acknowledge his body's cues for water, protein, and carbohydrates to power his workouts, and to recognize when his body said, "Stop." Meditation and relaxation developed into useful substitutes for combating out-of-control cravings to overeat.

Skill Builder: Decreasing Exercise Obsession

1. Consult a professional trainer. Ask that person to help you establish a routine, and stick to it. To stay honest, make a verbal commitment to a friend (or therapist) about your balanced, mindful exercise plan.

2. Study yourself. This self-study will focus on discovering your workout pattern. What prompts you to work out? Is it a feeling? A routine? To be healthy? For muscle development? What *function* does working out serve?

3. Find alternative ways to release stress in addition to working out.

4. Use low-impact substitutes. Go for walks. Do yoga. Stretch.

5. Experiment with the opposite of exercise. Relax. Rest. When you rest, be mindful of the experience.

6. If your body says, "Stop," don't ignore the warning. Your body sends your mind vital information for making decisions. Make informed choices.

7. If significant others, such as coaches or spouses, encourage you to overexercise, talk to them. Discuss your body's responses, your injuries, and your long-term physical goals.

8. Athletes are particularly vulnerable to overworking their bodies. Many believe that weight loss enhances performance. Although it may slightly maximize performance, that advantage will not last. Food fosters power, strength, and mental concentration. Consult a professional about your concerns to maximize your health and enhance your athletic performance.

26
Should You Clean Your Plate?

Healthy babies are incapable of overeating. Human beings, when they are born, know instinctively when they are hungry, and how to cry to alert others of their need to be fed. Babies stop eating when they are full. They cannot be forced to nurse or to finish a bottle when they have had enough. This suggests that there are biological sensors that dictate how much we should eat, and that overeating is, in part, a learned behavior.

One of the ways it may be learned is at the family dinner table. The parents of small children frequently demand that they "finish all the food on their plates." This sets up the behavior later in life of estimating how much to eat by how much is set in front of you, instead of eating as much as you need. This is a mindless approach.

If you always eat what is put in front of you, you are likely to be in trouble. Today, restaurant portions are out of control, and completely out of sync with mindful eating. Typically, supersized, gargantuan portions of restaurant food encourage mindless eating.

Susan became a mindful eater. When she went out to dinner she began to change how she figured out how much to eat. Instead of consuming everything on her plate, she noticed that she felt full after eating about two thirds of the portion, and when she felt full, she simply stopped eating. She also noticed that if she did eat everything on her plate, she became too full, which was the signal that she had not eaten mindfully.

Skill Builder: Mindfully Clean Your Plate!

Experiment with portion sizes. Instead of cleaning your entire plate, leave some food. See how your body responds. Listen to internal cues to know when to stop. When you are at restaurants, carefully measure how much you can comfortably eat without feeling any pressure to finish it all.

If you are an undereater and often intentionally leave most of your food uneaten, start listening to your inner dialogue about why you reject the food. Think about and try to feel whether it is your body or mind putting up the "Stop" sign. Eat until your stomach feels full. Pay attention to the signals your stomach sends, rather than listening to your mind generating self-critical thoughts.

Part III

Mindfulness of Feelings

By effort and heedfulness, discipline and self-mastery, let the wise one make for himself an island, which no flood can overwhelm.

—Buddha

27
Mindfully Cope with Emotional Eating

In reaction to every event, a feeling generally follows. Just like the urge we have to categorize and sort objects such as socks, bills, and money, we desire a simple and organized way to understand our feelings. As a result, people tend to classify even complex emotions into three simple categories: pleasant, unpleasant, or neutral.

Feelings, also called emotions, are a myriad of complex, confusing, constantly changing sensations that can flood and/or cloud your awareness. Feelings are like the weather, natural yet uncontrollable. The trick is to forecast storms of intense anger or irritability and the emptiness of a chilly, lonely day. Protect your inner climate from extreme conditions. Remember feelings come and go and evolve quickly, which demands a watchful and flexible eye. Therefore, do not react to them at their onset or before you understand what they are really about. Feelings are extremely transient. This is demonstrated by thinking about the way memory tends to work. For example, think about something that really upset you in the past. Today, it is more than likely that it doesn't bother you at all. You might even laugh about it. Just because you feel an emotion doesn't mean you have to do anything about it. Label your feelings. Name them, and you end their power over you by identifying them as "just feelings."

Use meditation to get in touch with your emotions. Identify which feelings you repeatedly experience before and after you eat. Are they shame, guilt, or disappointment? Is it a combination of these three? Think about how you cope with these feelings. Do they stop any further analysis of your behavior by paralyzing your ability to think? Are you aware of your judgments? Do you listen to how many times a day your mind translates "This food is bad for me" into "I'm a bad person?" Do you hear, "I ate really well today, so I'm a good person?" Stop waiting for your verdict about how you feel each time you eat, and become more aware of the process. This will help you to make wise choices about your eating, based on your nutritional needs as opposed to your feelings.

Skill Builder: Walking Backward and Forward

Meditation brings wisdom; lack of meditation leaves ignorance. Know well what leads you forward and what holds you back, and choose the path that leads to wisdom.

—Buddha

If you have had a period of mindless eating, think about what happened before it. Retrace your steps. Go over your experience backwards, and identify all of the individual steps that led to where you are now. Do it one step at a time.

1. Ask yourself this question. What began your mindless eating? What happened right before you started eating? Often, examining the context of the situation leads you back to the feelings and thoughts that prompted the situation. There are many factors that could have made you susceptible to uncontrolled eating.

2. After you walk through the incident backwards, walk through it again, going forwards this time. Be aware of the feelings that occurred after your bout of mindless eating.

3. Once you have walked through the incident, try to identify those points when you might have taken a different path. Commit the circumstances of this critical juncture to your memory.

Enduring and Controlling Difficult Moods

Mindless chaotic, over- and undereaters generally respond similarly to extreme feelings. Whether good or bad, intense emotions become overwhelming and often intolerable. In general, the wish is to *get rid of them* as soon as possible. Eating is one way to change or modulate emotions quickly. People use food to stuff down feelings, or they starve themselves and thus ward off feeling anything at all. People also use food to soothe, diminish, or intensify feelings. They use it to purge and release emotions, and to regain control over their moods.

Skill Builder: Don't Let Your Emotions Eat You Up

The following exercises will help you cope with difficult emotions in the moment rather than allowing them to eat you up.

1. Identify the feeling. Full awareness is always the key. Write a letter to yourself describing the emotion. Observe it first, then describe it.

2. Bump it down a notch. Imagine that you can quantify the level of your emotion, and adjust it, just as you can tune the dial that sets your radio volume. If you are at ten, make a plan about what needs to happen to reduce it to a six.

3. If you are feeling anxious, let your body go. Reconnect with your body. Feel your feet against the floor. Let your shoulders and neck drop. Observe how it feels not to resist the pull of gravity.

4. If you are feeling stressed, imagine giving yourself a body massage. Picture yourself lying on your stomach. First, focus on your feet and imagine them being massaged with scented oils. Be mindful of your ankles and calves as they are being rubbed. In your mind, allow the massage to travel down your neck, shoulders, arms, and fingertips. Imagine turning over on your stomach and feeling the kneading deep in the muscles of your lower back.

5. If you feel sad, be sad. Don't fight it. Rent a sad movie, call a friend and talk about it. Teach yourself that bad feelings aren't intolerable or scary. They can be accepted.

6. Anger is a particularly difficult emotion. It often occurs secondary to a primary emotion. Frustration, hurt, or fear of loss may be behind an angry feeling. Admit your anger and discover what is prompting it. Take a mental snapshot of the moment. Step back and take the same picture with a panoramic lens. What else is in the picture? Buddha said that, "Holding on to anger is like grasping a hot coal with the intent of throwing it at someone else; but you are the one who gets burned."

7. If you're feeling guilty, confess that to yourself. Admit you feel guilty. Remember that mindfulness is about being nonjudgmental. If you see yourself sentencing yourself to a punishment, think again. Handing out a punishment will only start another mindless eating cycle. You gain more power by being compassionate

with yourself, and your compassion will prevent negative feelings from arising that could trigger more mindless eating.

8. If you are feeling overwhelmed by emotions and, typically, you push them down, imagine you have a pressure valve somewhere on your body. Turn the knob slowly. Let out a little bit of emotion at a time. Remember, you are in charge of turning the handle.

9. Midday and/or end-of-the-day rituals. Observing rituals can be a helpful way to release emotions that build up throughout the day. Daily routines have a grounding effect and foster awareness. Write one page in your journal, sing a soothing song, burn incense, or repeat a prayer aloud. Try to do this at the same time every day. Practicing ritual is similar to the feelings you get when you hear a song you know well. It is familiar, uncomplicated, and you can predict how much you will like it.

10. If you feel as if you want to harm yourself, call 911. When you want to injure yourself, this means that the emotions you are experiencing are too intense for you to contain. Find a safe place with people who can help you moderate and understand your feelings.

Endurance is one of the most difficult disciplines, but it is to the one who endures that the final victory comes.

—Buddha

28
Mindful Metaphors—
Visualize Your Feelings

I am terrified of eating fat because I fear blowing up like a big, red beach ball. The kind of ball that people kick around, and let float away when they don't feel like it's worth rescuing out of deep water.

I feel skinless. Any kind of emotion feels like it is touching my raw nerve endings. When people look at me, I feel naked and unprotected. I want a porous emotional skin that lets people in, and protects me from being afraid they are evaluating my body.

These statements are two examples of the many vivid metaphors people create to describe the experience of mindless, problematic eating. Creating and describing analogies, parables, myths, stories, and personal anecdotes encourages people to look beyond the surface of their problems. Transforming your experience into an image or a poetic metaphor can help you step back and examine your problem from a different perspective.

For example, Kate battled her guilt about eating and her tortured thoughts about her body by visualizing a mindful eating metaphor. She compared her body's chronic fatigue, which she experienced from lack of calories, to a car sputtering to a stop because it's out of gas. She visualized herself as a little blue Volvo, and the food she ate as putting fuel in the tank. The busier she was, and the harder she pushed down on the pedal, the more often she had to fill the tank with quality gas (protein, complex carbohydrates), not the cheap gas (diet sodas, cookies, chips). Kate became more mindful of the way her body moved, and of its many critical functions like breathing and walking. She realized that if she was not mindful, she would be driving down a road that would crash and ruin her body.

Skill Builder: Creating Mindful Eating Metaphors

If you could describe what your eating issue looks like, what would you see? Think about its color, shape, and size. Would it be like an animal, person, place, or object? Once you have observed and described the image, you can begin to transform it into a more mindful image.

29
Control Your Feelings
with Your Nose

If you don't know how you feel, your breathing will tell you. Breathing reflects your emotions. If you are anxious, it is shallow and fast, if you are relaxed, it is slow and rhythmic. When you "hold" your breath, it is a strong clue that you are frightened. When in love, your breath is "taken away." Therefore, by paying attention to your breathing, you can become aware of your inner emotions. If you don't know what you are feeling, stop, pay attention to your breathing, and let your breathing help you tune into your feelings.

Skill Builder: Deep Breathing Before You Eat

For many people, eating is a stressful event. If this is so for you, sit down at the table and prepare yourself to be in a mindful state before you eat. Focus all of your attention on your bodily sensations. Relax and make yourself comfortable. Lean back in your chair and be aware of the position of your body. Relax your muscles, close your eyes, and let your body unwind. Tense and release your muscles. Begin by taking a deep breath. Very slowly, take a deep breath that allows your diaphragm to move up and down. Concentrate on the sound of your breath. Listen to it and feel the sensations as you breathe. Feel yourself relax as the tension releases and leaves your body. Follow the journey of the air as it travels through your nose and throat, fills up your lungs, and moves your chest. Take just a moment to connect with your breathing as you gear up to eat mindfully.

30
How Much Do You Weigh (Psychologically)?

At times, a scale becomes not only the measure of your weight but the measure of your worth, and a strong determinant of your mood and well-being. Unfortunately, when this happens, you turn over your sense of control to something outside of yourself. When the scale presents you with a number you don't like, you may judge yourself too harshly. This can jeopardize your balance because you become dominated or literally weighed down by your self-critical judgments. Rather than judging yourself, it would be more helpful to think about weighing yourself psychologically.

Skill Builder: Weighing Your Self-Esteem

Meditate on how much appetite and food problems weigh you down. Work more on diminishing the weight of other stresses in your life than on your gravitational physical weight. Your self-esteem is comprised of several components. Think about how you feel about yourself intellectually, morally, physically, socially, economically, and spiritually. Which aspect of your self is most out of balance and tipping your scales? Now, think about those times in your life when you felt good about yourself. Make sure you identify times that aren't related to your body or physical appearance. Consider what you can do to feel good about yourself that is not related to eating or to your weight.

31
Mindful Eating and Relationships

The quality and depth of your relationships with the important people in your life are often good indicators of, and parallel to, your relationship with food. It can be useful to think about your interactions with food using "relationship" terms, because eating is an inescapable part of your daily routine. You make decisions every day about how much priority and attention to give to food in ways that may be similar to how you balance the priorities and attention you give to partners, family, and friends. The way you eat may reflect the nature of your relationships with people. For example, if you are a chronic dieter and you feel your worth is inseparable from your weight, your relationships may not have much depth. Or, if you restrict and avoid certain foods, your relationships are more likely to be more superficial, sometimes even one-dimensional, which leaves you feeling isolated and disconnected.

For example, Janet described her relationship to food to be like that of a defendant in a continual "court trial." With each bite, she felt compelled to present all the nutritional reasons why she "should" be allowed to eat it, in order to convince the invisible jury in her head that she wouldn't become fat from eating it. She interacted with friends in a suspiciously similar manner. Janet felt guilty saying "no" to anyone, and spent agonizing hours trying to make a simple decision about going somewhere with a friend.

Skill Builder: Stop Food Fights

Be mindful of the significance of food in your life and how that also may describe your relationships. How would you characterize your relationship to food? Is it a secret love affair occurring in quiet, hidden places? Do you keep your food and eating habits a secret from those around you? Or, is it a love/hate relationship? Do the foods you crave lead you to despise yourself after you have surrendered to their pleasure? Is food a reliable "friend" when you need it, or a constant "enemy" you try to avoid and/or conquer? Describe your current relationship with food, and think about the kind of relationship you would like it to become. Aim for a friendship or partnership that is even, fair, open to communication, and constantly negotiating the competing needs of your body and mind.

Relationships May Trigger Mindless Eating

Buddha said, "An insincere and evil friend is to be more feared than a wild beast; a wild beast may wound your body, but an evil friend will wound your mind." This saying succinctly captures how harmful a bad relationship can be to your state of mind and sense of well-being. Interpersonal problems are notoriously guilty of limiting one's ability to live and act mindfully. People can become caught in constant worry about the state of their relationships. Questions like, "Do people like me?" and "What do they think of me?" may be in the forefront of your mind. Relationship difficulties can consume you, and keep you from focusing on the task at hand, which is being present for the important people in your life and really enjoying life.

One frequently asked question goes, "If my body isn't really attractive, will people like me?" It is true that many people often make their first judgments based on appearances. But real relationships are based on far more substantial connections. When you are truly mindful of your relationships, you examine people from a *holistic* approach. You are appreciative of all aspects of who they are. Mindfulness doesn't value anyone because of their past or future. Rather, it values people for who they are in the present moment. Get in touch with your reactions, and with what you "sense" and "feel" in a friend's presence, as opposed to what you "know" about him or her in the past, or think about who he/she will be in the future.

People with eating issues are often people pleasers. People pleasers care a lot about making others happy, often at the expense of their own well-being. People pleasing inhibits mindfulness because you are always anticipating how people will react as opposed to being fully present, and making decisions based on what you sense and feel in the moment, instead of thinking things through.

Skill Builder: Relationship Check

1. If you worry about what other people think about your body, start by evaluating the quality of your relationships. Do you judge other people exclusively on their appearance? If you are critical of yourself, do you "project" this onto other people and assume this is what they think about you? Consider how this might affect your relationships. What is it that you are afraid others will see if they really know you?

2. When you are with people, really be with them. Look in their eyes, touch their hands, keep your mind focused on the conversation. Take note of the feelings and thoughts that arise for you.

Skill Builder: Mindful Body Talk

1. Be more aware of the messages you receive and send to your friends. The Buddha said, "Thousands of candles can be lighted from a single candle, and the life of the candle will not be shortened. Happiness never decreases by being shared." Don't make fat-phobic

comments, check out others' bodies, or snicker about others' weight. Refuse to engage in disparaging talk about someone else's looks. When you find yourself giving someone the once-over and you make a critical comment, counter it with a positive observation. Genuinely compliment others.

2. Never, never, never comment on anyone's weight. You don't know what your comment may mean to someone, and you have no idea what kind of effect your comment may have on that person. Mindless eaters repeatedly report that other people's comments (both positive and negative) about their weight dramatically sway their eating habits. Unhealthy, even dangerous, mindless undereating is reinforced by well-meaning loved ones and coworkers saying, "Oh you look so thin," or "You don't need to lose weight." If you must say something, use a generalized compliment like, "You look really nice today." Don't emphasize weight. Saying that someone looks "fat" or has "gained weight" can be very cruel. Value people not for their butts, thighs, or stomachs, but for their hearts and minds.

32
Heart versus Hunger Cravings

Marie had one desire for St. Valentine's Day. She wanted to receive a large, red velvet heart full of chocolates. Days before the holiday she waited, craving the gift and imagining how pretty the box would be. Ironically, because of a mild food allergy, she didn't even like chocolate, and rarely ate it. Marie didn't realize that it wasn't chocolate she hungered for, but what the large, red heart symbolized. She wanted to be loved, and for her lover to express his love with a symbolic gift. This anecdote illustrates the kind of confusion that can exist between what your heart longs for and what your stomach craves.

Buddhist theory identifies cravings as the root of suffering. Emotional cravings can be more powerful, insatiable, and destructive than physical hunger. Your emotional desires aren't as clear-cut or as predictable as your desire to eat. As you become more mindful, you will begin to realize exactly what your heart hungers for. Examples include cravings for companionship, love, power, and control. In contrast to food, these longings are not as easily fulfilled. Sometimes, people misinterpret their heart cravings, and try to feed their bodies when they actually need to take better care of their souls.

For example, before Jessica became a mindful eater she was particularly vulnerable to overeating when lonely or sad. Now, instead of reaching for food as comfort, she mindfully calls a friend. It feels so good to talk to others that she stops thinking about overeating and rejoices in companionship.

Skill Builder: Keep a Mindfulness Journal

Keep track of your constantly changing emotions and desires. Carry a small pocket journal with you wherever you go. Make it easily accessible so you can reach it in the moment you experience fleeting, powerful, intense emotions or cravings. Or, buy a daily calendar that breaks down the day by hour. Jot down the emotions you felt at particular hours. Examine the calendar at the end of the day to see whether any patterns or trends emerge. If you spend most of your time in front of a computer, create an easily accessible, secure document file to record what happens to you emotionally when your mind wanders during the day.

In addition to your feelings, record and examine your daydreams. These can give you a good idea of what you are consciously craving. If you imagine a special relationship, you are likely craving love and attention. If you dream about a job promotion, you may be longing for power, control, and intellectual stimulation. Consider what you can do to satisfy your heart's cravings.

33
Mindful Holiday Feasting

Most people look forward to the joy of traditional holiday feasts. They are times of celebration for everyone, except mindless eaters. For mindless eaters, gatherings centered exclusively around food can turn not-so-merry. Worry about gaining extra holiday pounds is nothing to celebrate. Holidays elevate feasting to a special status, and they encourage mindless eating by inviting all to overeat.

Spending time with relatives during holidays is another surefire way to trigger mindless eating. Reconnecting with family can be as stressful as it is joyous. People get very emotional, and conflict is more likely to erupt. Hanging out with your family can reignite feelings of inadequacy or of being controlled, rejected, or wanting to please. Or, it may bring up intense memories of happy holidays from the past, which can make you miss more regular contact with your family. One woman described the Christmas holidays as the ultimate challenge because they are a double-dose of her two weaknesses: family and food.

Skill Builder: Planning Holiday Meals

- Plan ahead mindfully. Think about which foods define the holiday for you. Plan to have some of that special food. Offer to prepare the meal to have greater control over the menu. Make foods that don't trigger or increase your vulnerability to mindless eating.

- If the holiday meal is to be eaten at someone else's home, eat a mindful snack before you go. Don't wait until after the football game or holiday parade. If you do, your body will send you hunger cues that may be difficult to satiate in a controlled manner.

- Be mindful of unique ethnic and cultural traditions.

- If you are a chronic undereater, holidays can be extremely difficult. Reach back in your memory and identify what you liked to eat before your eating issues began. Eat what would make you happy. Connect yourself with the meaning of the holiday; for example, if it is the Fourth of July, celebrate the liberty you have to choose your foods.

- To prevent overeating, stay in touch with the experience moment-to-moment. At the table, eat slowly and look at everything. Smell and taste your food. Breathe in the holiday atmosphere.

- After finishing your plate, wait twenty minutes before getting a second helping. It takes the part of your brain that helps to regulate your appetite, about twenty minutes to register what you ate, and to send the information that you are full to your body and brain. Allow your body and mind the necessary time to send and receive these signals.

- If the same food is prepared in different ways, choose your favorite. For example, if there are mashed potatoes and sweet potatoes, consider which will give you the most pleasure, or have a small amount of both.

- If you have trouble knowing how much you have eaten, put the food on your plate in piles that don't overlap. Start with this, and then wait and see how your body responds.

34
Mindful Dining Out

Depending on your relationship to food, eating out can either be a special treat or a nightmare. Jill, for example, loved interesting, quaint cafés and was a regular at many local Thai restaurants. She didn't have to cook, and the flavor far surpassed anything she could create. The dark side of eating out was worrying about the excess calories. She had no control over how the food was prepared, and didn't know how many calories she was consuming, so she felt guilty. When she dined out as a reward to herself, she mindlessly overate. Eating out was a mixture of intense pleasure and equally intense remorse.

If dining out is a special event for you, that doesn't give you permission to eat mindlessly. Attentive, aware, nonjudgmental eating can take place anywhere. You can eat mindfully at restaurants exactly the way you do at home, by eating slowly and savoring your food. Learn to think of the restaurant's ambience and service as the real treat, rather than the food. Going out to eat is often a form of entertainment or a social event. Sometimes you may feel forced to choose between being social or engaging in mindless eating. However, the two need not be mutually exclusive. If dining out with friends brings up negative feelings, or causes you stress, be mindful of what's behind your concern. Your fear may cause you to assume that you will lose control. To combat the fear, use it as an opportunity to be mindful of your relationships, and to practice your mindful eating skills.

Food comparison is a common but disturbing phenomenon that people must deal with when eating with friends. Food comparers place their orders based on what other people are eating. This is an example of mindless eating because it is more mindful of someone else's behavior than your own. Both your experience of and relationship to food are uniquely yours. For this reason, it is important for you to focus and meditate on your own experience. Eat from your own plate.

Skill Builder: Eleven Ways to Dine Out

1. The first step in planning an evening out is to choose a restaurant mindfully. This means picking one with a large selection of healthy, interesting foods. Avoid buffet style, "All You Can Eat," one-price, three-course meals, or places with limited selections. This falls under the same set of rules as avoiding the grocery store when hungry.

2. To help avoid mindless eating, have a small snack before you go. Don't go really hungry, and don't "save up" calories for this meal. When you are moderately hungry as opposed to very hungry, it is much easier to make mindful choices and to refuse food you normally wouldn't eat. Very hungry people are likely to eat anything put in front of them. Moderately hungry people are choosier. If you are really hungry, you will likely order too much. To avoid overeating, choose something similar to what you would prepare at home. Eat slowly and savor the entire experience.

3. Eat mindfully and stay attuned to your relationships with people and with food. Talk, laugh, and have a good time. If you are attacked by guilt-ridden thoughts about eating, keep your eyes and 90 percent of your attention on the people with you.

4. If you are a "food comparer" or are competitive about your weight, order first so you won't be tempted to change your pick. Focus on positive food talk.

Compliment the taste. Don't join with others if they are engaging in hypercritical food talk. Consider not dining out with people who raise your anxiety level or with people who are overly focused on their own eating issues. Find people who are good, mindful eating role models.

5. Become more relationship-focused by ordering together and sharing the food. If you are hungry for a particular food that is normally off-limits for you, such as an appetizer or a dessert, ask someone at your table to share half of an order with you. Sharing exotic food can be fun. Make a joint decision about your pick. Discuss your likes and dislikes rather than dwelling on food that you can't have. Have fun. Enjoy your meal.

6. Do not judge what others eat. No one wants to dine with someone who criticizes their food choices. If someone chooses greasy French fries that you wouldn't dare touch, be aware of your reaction. Say to yourself, "I'm judging and I need to be more compassionate. I notice that I become envious and critical at the same time. I need to focus on my eating and my eating alone." At other times, you might feel guilty that your "thinner" companion is eating less than you are. Again, be mindful of your needs and everything going on within yourself.

7. Minimize using food as a way to celebrate or provide pleasure. Buy a gift, send a card, leave a very thoughtful voice-mail message. Sometimes people joke about needing a "chocolate fix" to mend the strains of a stressful day. You know that in the long run, food just won't do it. Reinforcing the notion that food provides the ultimate comfort is just plain dangerous.

8. Don't make a show of what you order. Sometimes people like to get validation (or an envious reaction) by ordering their meal to be served without cheese, oil, butter, etc. Give the waitperson your order based on your taste preferences, not to provoke a reaction.

9. Avoid picking at your food mindlessly. When bread is brought to your table, take a piece or two, and send the rest away. Bread (and butter) are among the most common mindlessly eaten foods. Also, when you are done with your meal, move your plate to the side, or ask to have it removed. It's easy to put more food on your plate mindlessly, or pick at it when it is in front of you.

10. Loosen the connection between eating and socializing. If your friends ask you out to dinner frequently, suggest meeting for coffee or tea instead. Plan non-food-related activities like walks or movies. Or, invite your friends to a dinner you will prepare.

11. Don't conduct business meetings or important discussions over a meal. It is difficult to be attentive to your eating when you must engage in critical or emotional conversation at the table. People tend to use food unconsciously to soothe tension.

35
Accept Your Genes

Betsy's family joked that she, like other women in the family, had been cursed with the "Cervellonis' hips." The women on her father's side all had wide, sturdy hips and buttocks that were a painful contrast to the thin, elegant hips and dainty butt that she fantasized about when she worked out. When she examined her family lineage, it was clear that her desire to fit into size six pants was unrealistic. No matter how much she dieted and worked out, her bone structure and her body type would not change. Also, if your family members have difficulty modulating their eating, unfortunately, it is likely that you, too, will also have to struggle to modulate your eating.

Body shape and weight range are largely influenced by genetics. Your bone size, metabolism rate, and fat deposit locations are determined by your genetic code as much as your eye, hair color, and height are.

According to the "set point" theory, it is postulated that your body has a genetically predetermined weight range. Your body tries to keep your weight within that range and will automatically adjust your metabolism and food storage capacity to keep you from losing or gaining weight outside of that range or set point. The set point theory suggests that little can be done to change your overall body shape in the same way that your shoe size, height, and eye color are a predetermined part of who you are. All you can do to alter this is to tint your contacts and wear high-heeled shoes. Similarly, you can subtly alter the appearance of your body shape by the clothes you wear, or by toning your muscles with exercise.

Angie, for example, was five feet, three inches tall. Her weight fell naturally within a range of 115–125 pounds. If she ate mindfully, her body weight stayed comfortably within this range. She noticed that it was extremely difficult to lose any weight if she weighed 115 pounds, and her body felt uncomfortable when it broached the upper limit. Angie's ability to listen to her body helped her to eat mindfully and to stay within her natural range.

Skill Builder: Identify Your Natural Body Shape

Draw a family tree. Identify those family members who have struggled with mindless eating. If food and weight haven't been a topic of conversation, look at family pictures. Take into account how bodies changed from childhood to old age. Think about whether over-, under-, or chaotic eating is a family pattern. While you are at it, appreciate the family traits that people admire and compliment, like unique green eyes or naturally curly hair.

Adopted Families and Food Anxiety

If you were adopted or frequently ate with people other than your biological parents, your primary caregivers still played a significant role in shaping your eating habits. They did this by what they fed you and the messages about food they taught to you. Linda's adoptive mother provides a poignant example of how subtle, mindless eating habits are learned. Although Linda's mother did not encourage her daughter to diet, she constantly restricted her own food intake. She never ate the elaborate meals she prepared for her family. Linda observed her mother's eating habits and subconsciously incorporated them into her own routines. She wouldn't eat foods her mom avoided because they had "too much fat." Never underestimate the importance of your environment and role models.

Skill Builder: Identify Learned Food Habits

Write a list of what constituted a "typical meal" when you were growing up. List how many times a day you ate, and what the common foods and snacks were. What kind of messages did you receive about your body, food, and how to eat as a child and adolescent? How do those messages affect you now? What kind of food culture do you want to create in your own family, dorm, or household?

36
Change Mindless Eating Traps

Mindless eating is more likely to occur in the same place, over and over again. To make life simpler, the mind takes advantage of any shortcuts it can. For example, when looking for underwear, your hand will automatically go to your underwear drawer. If you rearrange your drawers and put your underwear in a new location, your hand will still tend to travel automatically to the old drawer, until new shortcuts are formed in your brain. We make connections between events and we have to work hard to break and form new links.

If you practice mindless eating in certain places, your brain is likely to subconsciously remember that and act out of habit. Never, under any circumstances, eat in front of the TV, computer screen, while driving, or on the phone. These are the most notorious locations for mindless eating. Jessica's vulnerable spot was in her kitchen. To take control, Jessica created a mindful eating haven in her home. This was away from the refrigerator, phone, TV, and other distractions. Before eating, she put all the food portions she planned to eat on the table, so she would not have to return to the kitchen. She learned to relax and breathe between each bite, and to watch herself in the process of eating. This slowed her down enough to enjoy her meals in a mindful way.

Cafeteria-style dining encourages uncontrolled, unaware eating. The unstructured abundance of food is a dangerous place for automatic, mindless eating. Instead of choosing what is appealing, choices are often based on thoughts like, "I want to get my money's worth," or "I want to try everything." For overeaters, buffets are an overwhelming sea of choices. Mindless undereaters also find buffets difficult. To cope, they eat only their familiar foods rather than trying anything new. For under-, over-, and chaotic eaters, the anxiety caused by too much food can supercede any enjoyment a buffet might offer. It is wise not to go to them before you have mindless eating skills down pat.

Skill Builder: Pinpoint Your Mindless Eating Cues

Learn which situations tend to act as the cues that entice you to eat without thoughtfulness. Identify the places you are most likely to eat mindlessly. In the kitchen, at the local coffee shop, at your desk? Find ways to turn a space in your environment into a place that fosters mindful eating. In that place, remove any clutter that could distract you while you eat. Objects like phones or clocks that pull you away from a mindful state should be moved elsewhere.

Put your place setting so that it faces away from the kitchen (or refrigerator). Bring food to the table before you eat, so you won't have to get up. Or, create a new space. Tailor it to be a calm, peaceful environment that brings you to a mindful state. If you wish, burn incense or change the lighting. Add a pretty tablecloth and fresh flowers. Play soothing music. Hang up a sign in your danger area that says, "Eat Mindfully" to realert you to your mindful stance.

37
Filling Up on Fun

Unfortunately, boredom and/or a feeling of emptiness are very common reasons that people eat when they are not hungry. Eating, or continuously thinking about eating, fills up a stretch of time and can feel purposeful. The emptiness of being alone can be as painful as a hollow stomach. If thinking about eating takes over a significant amount of your day, you may want to consider reorganizing your energy. Be mindful of other activities that will satisfy you as much as food does, and feed your soul, as well.

Skill Builder: Boredom Blockers

Make a list of activities that will keep you from turning to food or thoughts of food in downtimes. Remember, *"A generous heart, kind speech, and compassionate service to others are renewing forces."* Be actively aware, awake, and moving. Mindfully go shopping, read, participate in hobbies and sports, call someone, take a nap. Write in your journal. Turn your thoughts to being mindful of others. By far, the best way to fill your heart and mind is to spend time with caring friends. Whatever you choose to do, feed your mind by participating actively in the world.

38
Mindfully Imperfect

Julie didn't think she had any food issues or problems. She was a perfectionist, and, on the surface, everything in her life seemed to be perfect. Except it wasn't. She had received stellar grades in school, found an excellent job, and won the admiration of her peers. But she was constantly unhappy about her body, and practiced never-ending self-disapproval. Her self-criticism plagued her thoughts and prevented her from appreciating all that she had accomplished.

Feeling bad about yourself is a common source of mindless eating. A poor self-image usually begins early in life and is fostered by a variety of life experiences. Acting "perfectly" often results in attention, validation, and praise. Whether it's straight A's, or a toned body, living up to extremely high standards is praised and envied by others. This can create the illusion that everything is okay. But the consequences of trying to live up to unrealistically high standards for your body are that you may spend your life in misery, and believe you are a "failure," despite whatever else you accomplish.

If you look beneath your obsessive concerns about your appearance, you may find that you really fear the possibility that you are not "good" enough or "smart" enough or "interesting enough" to win others' interest or approval. Or you may find that you don't want to let others into your life at all. You can hide more easily behind a "perfect" appearance. Having a great body is one aspect of seeming to "have it all together." Typically, perfectionism in any area of your life may intensify your desire to have a "perfect body." But the need for perfection can be a trap that keeps you from enjoying your life and being proud of your accomplishments.

Skill Builder: Striving for Mindful Imperfection

Are you a perfectionist? Do you catch yourself saying things to yourself (or others) like "I'm not good enough" or "People won't like me if I make mistakes," or "I have to be the very best"? Think about where such unrealistic expectations of yourself originated. Did your parents pressure you to succeed, or is this need to be the best self-inflicted? To feel good about yourself, do you depend on praise from others?

1. If you answered "yes" to the questions above, consider the "cost" of perfectionism, particularly in terms of your heath, and the wear and tear of stress on your emotional well-being. Learn how to weigh the costs and benefits of doing your best as opposed to striving for unobtainable perfection.

2. Develop a list of your expectations and goals. Evaluate how "realistic" each one is.

3. Intentionally do something imperfectly on a small scale, and evaluate what happens.

4. Be mindful of the processes, instead of the outcomes.

5. If you feel you've "messed up" or had a difficult eating day, remember the broader scope of your life. Make a list of your positive qualities and achievements (finishing your degree, your talent for writing, taking care of your two babies, the way you care for other people, etc.). This may sound like a simplistic, trite exercise, but sometimes, when you feel as if nothing is going right for you, you may need a tangible reminder that you are okay and that you've accomplished a lot in your life.

After you make your list, hang it up where you can see it when you need it. When you are sad and blue, it is easier to wallow in negatives than to remember the positives about yourself. If you can't identify your own positives, make a list with a friend. Or, create a list for each other. Give a copy to your friend and call him or her when you need a reminder from the outside world. Someone who can remind you of your strengths should be a treasured friend.

Part IV

Mindfulness of Thoughts

The thought manifests as the word; the word manifests as the deed; the deed develops into habit; and habit hardens into character. So watch the thought and its ways with care, and let it spring from love born out of concern for all beings.

—Buddha

39
Changing Mindless Thinking

Mindless thinking is like looking into a fun house mirror. Because of a flaw in the glass, the mirror cannot reflect a true image. The way the mirror is distorted makes it impossible to see what you really look like. People with eating issues are plagued with distorted thinking patterns that are similar to the distortions of fun house mirrors. The way mindless thinking works makes it impossible to evaluate situations wisely. The consequence of mindless thinking is that it unconsciously affects your eating habits. Identifying the presence of these distorted thoughts in your head is the first step toward taking away their power.

Mindless eaters tend to get stuck in extreme thinking patterns. It's similar to getting your car stuck in the mud. The more you turn the wheel in the same way, the deeper the car will sink. When closely examined, the logic of mindless eaters is often influenced by skewed perceptions, over and over again. In contrast, those who follow The Middle Way think temperate, moderate thoughts that are in the moment, observant, nonjudgmental, and accepting.

The following sections describe nine types of mindless thinking. They also describe how The Middle Way would deal with the issues.

1. **Extreme Thinking:** This consists of "either"/or" thoughts. They don't allow any room for a middle ground or gray area. *Examples:* "I am either perfect or I am a failure," "I am either beautiful or I am ugly." The Middle Way would say, "I may not be happy with every aspect of my body, but I am not ugly. There are many things I like about my body and myself. There are some things I do not."

2. **Worst Case Scenario:** This is the mental habit of overgeneralizing the potential outcome of a situation. *Example:* "If I eat this cookie, I will gain ten pounds, and no one will ever want to go out with me again." The Middle Way would say, "I will not gain weight if I eat this cookie. I am trying to eat moderately to feel better about myself. People like me for many other reasons besides my body."

3. **Overstating the Facts:** This consists of sweeping statements that use one rule and apply it to a number of situations. *Example:* "Being fat means you must be lazy." The Middle Way would say, "Being overweight does not imply anything about my energy or my personality. That is a judgmental, mindless thought."

4. **Turning the Micro into Macro:** This mental habit blows up the importance of an issue to gargantuan proportions. *Example:* "If I purge again, my life will be ruined forever." The Middle Way would say, "I don't like it when I purge my food. It is very hard on my body, and I feel bad after I do it."

5. **Abracadabra Thoughts:** These consist of superstitious beliefs that seem to hold special powers. *Example:* "If I run three miles a day, I will not gain weight." The Middle Way would say, "How much weight I lose depends on many different factors. I want to exercise to be healthy."

6. **Putting on the Blinders:** This takes place when you ignore important information. *Example:* "I don't see any evidence of physical problems, so my doctor must be wrong. The way I eat is not harmful to me." The Middle Way would say, "I know mindless eating is not good for my body. Although I was uncomfortable when my doctor pointed this out, I realize the impact

unhealthy eating can have over the long run, and I am aware of the consequences."

7. **Overdoing It:** These are thoughts that blow up one's importance or relevance to a situation. *Example:* "Everyone is looking at my body. They are all laughing at me." The Middle Way would say, "I am exaggerating. I am feeling quite vulnerable right now. A glance is just a glance."

8. **Random Theories:** These are personal theories developed from faulty thoughts. *Example:* "If I purge my food, I will feel relieved. So, if I continue to purge, I will never feel distressed again." The Middle Way would say, "There are lots of things besides purging that help me feel relaxed. It's not the only way."

9. **No Back Up:** These are assumptions that are made without any concrete evidence to support them. *Example:* "People always like those who are thin and exercise a lot." The Middle Way would say, "I would like this to be true because it would help me feel more in control. However, I know I don't like everyone who is thin and exercises a lot. Therefore, this must not be true."

Skill Builder: Observing and Healing Mindless Thoughts

Identify which types of mindless thinking you practice frequently. When you catch yourself thinking in any of these ways, say to yourself, "That is an example of an "extreme thought" or [fill in the blank _____], and it is affecting what I decide to eat." Then, ask yourself, "If I followed The Middle Way, how would that thought be phrased?"

40
Impartial Thoughts

You may be surprised to learn that you label and categorize major parts of your eating behavior. Obviously, negative, self-punishing labels are harmful. However, positive phrases like, "I'm eating right" or "I am a good person for resisting potato chips" are also detrimental. Any words with either pleasant or critical connotations distract from just being mindful of the experience. Positive and negative words either reinforce or punish, which can increase or decrease the probability of a behavior reoccurring.

Resisting a handful of potato chips may be an example either of mindful or mindless eating depending on a variety of factors, such as how hungry you are or whether eating the potato chips is in the context of a binge. Clearly, the same item of food may be considered "good" at one time and "bad" at another. The key to mindful eating is to evaluate correctly whether the food you contemplate eating is the food you need (and want) in that moment without judgment.

Eating that isn't evaluated as "good" or "bad" is "neutral" and therefore tends to slip out of your awareness. Fruits and vegetables are most often neutral foods. Typically, eating an apple produces few to no emotions. If you are eating an apple mindfully, you are more likely to think about its juiciness, crunchiness, and tartness than your feelings. Such "neutral" experiences of eating clearly demonstrate that it is possible to eat without experiencing shameful, guilt-ridden emotions.

Skill Builder: Think About Food Impartially

Think about and identify which foods tend to escape your awareness when you eat them. Becoming mindful of the way you categorize foods as good, bad, and neutral will demonstrate to you that your judgments about eating and your emotions are tightly intertwined. Strive to think about food in a nonjudgmental, impartial way.

41
Mindful Imagery

Imagining a successful outcome is essential to changing any kind of behavior. Often, people unconsciously get stuck in expecting, and they fixate on failure. According to the psychological principle of "self-fulfilling prophecies," your behavior unconsciously leads you right down the path toward what you are expecting. If you expect to fail, you will unknowingly act in ways that make failure more likely. The opposite is equally true. If you expect to succeed, then imagery can help you succeed.

Using imagery, you can step back from the experience and imagine a healthy, desirable outcome. In Buddha's words, "He is able who thinks he is able." This skill values the power of thinking positive thoughts.

Skill Building: Using Guided Imagery

Choose one example of mindless eating that you struggle with routinely. For example, going out to dinner is often an experience people "expect" to fail. This is both unfortunate and unnecessary. Using guided imagery can be helpful for anticipating challenging feelings. Furthermore, it can guide you to identifying the factors that threaten your mindfulness.

Breathe slowly and deeply in and out. Close your eyes and continue to breathe from your diaphragm. Imagine walking into your favorite Italian restaurant. As you enter, you begin to pick up the mouthwatering odors of garlic and spices. Breathe them in and out. Focus on your breathing and your senses. Relax. Look around the restaurant. Imagine sitting down at a table. The tablecloth is a checkered red and white pattern. There is a long, red candle stuck in an empty wine bottle. It is lit. Watch the flame flicker. In the background, you hear soft Italian music. Focus on how you're feeling. Be in touch with all of your senses.

The waiter comes to your table and hands you a menu. As you open it, check out your feelings. What are they? Name them to yourself. Your eyes scan the menu for something that entices you. What thoughts come to mind? Label them as just thoughts. What feelings flow in and out of your consciousness? Do you feel overwhelmed by the choices, or guilty for desiring a certain food? Focus on your feelings and your breathing.

Now, imagine the food you want to eat arriving at your table. Examine the dish you ordered. Describe what it smells like, the texture, and the taste. How does it feel in your mouth, against your tongue, teeth, lips, as it travels to your stomach? Imagine eating this meal with all your mindful skills in place: observing, accepting, nonjudgmental, and aware of any clinging to the thought of failure. How does it feel within your body? Stay with every emotion that comes up for you. Name those emotions.

42
Mindful Realism

Mindfulness encourages you to eat what works well in your life, rather than what you *think* is "right" or "correct." Mindfulness doesn't strive for a particular result or require a specific change. We often do this by arbitrarily picking a number to be a weight goal. In fact, it doesn't dictate anything you should or should not do, because that boils down to making a judgment. Thus, be suspicious of diets professing to be the "only" way to lose weight. There are many strategies for controlling your eating habits. Food myths and fad diets all profess to know what is "right" to eat, but, unfortunately, they all contradict each other. Also, it is easy to think more about the future outcome of mindful eating than it is to think about what will help you to eat mindfully. When you spend a great deal of time fantasizing about your "ideal" weight, also ask yourself whether you can handle the dramatic changes you are contemplating, or what kinds of steps you need to take to reach your goal. Is losing ten pounds worth the daily aggravation, limitations on your lifestyle, and stress on your body?

Any strategy that helps you to eat mindfully, provided that it is nutritious and realistic, can be employed. When people choose diets and foods they don't like, or that aren't compatible with their lifestyle, those diets and foods simply won't work. The key is knowing yourself well. This will help you to identify what is *doable*, *safe*, and *pragmatic*.

For example, Stacy had struggled with problematic eating for more than ten years. She frequently binged on junk food for hours at a time. Mostly, she ate out of boredom and loneliness. Regardless of numerous diets and attempts at therapy, once she began eating, she was unable to leave the kitchen. One day, while she was bingeing, her dog, Mickey, her long-time companion, sat at her feet and looked up at her. According to Stacy, the look in Mickey's eyes said to her, "Why are you doing this to yourself? I care about you and don't want to see you go through this." At that point, Stacy put down the food, left the kitchen, and took Mickey for a walk. During the walk, she focused and meditated on the sense of peacefulness she felt. Thereafter, whenever she had the urge to binge, she took Mickey for a walk around the block. You won't find any documented "Walk Your Dog" methods to control your eating in any diet books. Nevertheless, walking her dog worked for Stacy.

Mindful behavior becomes obvious when you focus less on goals and critical "shoulds" and "shouldn'ts," and more on an awareness of what works.

Skill Builder: Your Personal Food Myths

1. Make a list of your food myths. These are the behaviors that you believe you "should" be doing. For example, one food myth is that all sweets are "bad" and should be strictly avoided. After listing your "right" and "wrong" food myths, transform these into mindful attitudes that are realistic and likely to work. A more realistic stance in this example might be eating that eating *too many* sweets is unhealthy, but eating an occasional, moderately portioned dessert is a more realistic, pragmatic, and doable stance.

2. It is important to consult a nutritionist about your perceived food myths. When you have become entangled in mindless eating, it may be hard to know whether your nutritional knowledge is on target or skewed. One woman felt very guilty after eating a small bowlful of carrots. She defined this as

overeating. Although carrots are healthy vegetables, a "small bowlful" of anything seemed wrong. Her mind had lost the ability to observe her behavior in a realistic manner.

3. It may also be necessary to seek a second opinion because everyone has been inundated with misinformation about nutrition. For example, one commonly held belief holds that all fat is bad. But some types of fat in your diet are essential for good health. Protecting internal organs, transporting vitamins, making hormones, providing energy, and forming parts of your brain and nervous system are just a few examples of the vital functions that fat performs.

43
Mindfully Adapting

Mindfulness is not about trying to change yourself. Instead, as you get more in touch with yourself, changes will happen naturally in positive ways, and they will be in tune with your body's emotional and physical needs. When you understand and are in touch with how your body responds to the way you feed it, you will adapt your eating in a natural way. Do not make drastic changes to your diet. Small steps in the right direction make a significant difference over time. Changing just one behavior can have a huge overall impact.

Learning to become mindful is a way of thinking that develops over time. Instead of saying a task has been done "well" or "poorly," we think of it as having been done in a "skillful" or "unskillful" manner. This acknowledges individual abilities, and recognizes that what is right for one person may not be so for another. Also, it is critical to remember that learning how to eat mindfully is a gradual *process*. It can be likened to earning different belt colors when learning a martial art. The skills build upon each other. You start at the beginning wearing a white belt, and you earn new belt colors by mastering different sets of skills. The black belt is the goal signifying mastery, but the beginner works slowly through a variety of different belt colors before achieving that goal.

Skill Builder: Mindful Practice

Being mindful requires time and practice. It takes a conscious effort to be aware of the way you subconsciously interface with the world. Don't rush your practice. Take your time. Be mindful about learning mindfulness. You can use mindful techniques in every action, no matter how ordinary.

Open your eyes to experiences you didn't notice before. Choose a small task such as washing the dishes, often a distasteful job. Slow down the process. Don't think of it as an annoying chore but as a moment in your life that you embrace. Fall in love with the mundane tasks in life. When you begin to practice mindfulness skills, think about whether you are doing them in a skilled manner. Define specifically what acting "skillfully" means to you.

44
Thinking Out Mindful Meals

Full concentration is essential to achieve mindfulness. Buddha identified five "hindrances" that frequently block clear thinking. Greed, laziness, ill will, worry, and doubt often stand in the way of mindful awareness. These states cloud and complicate pure attentiveness. One very common "hindrance" to straightforward, peaceful mindful eating is inconsistency in your eating patterns.

Vicky, for example, fell into a vicious cycle of skipping breakfast and then overeating at lunch. Eliminating her calorie intake in the morning served only to make her ravenously hungry at midday. She made unwise, out-of-control choices at lunch because she believed she had room to "make up for" the calories she had missed at breakfast. The result was that she ended up eating more calories than she would have if she had had a sensible breakfast and been only moderately hungry at lunch.

As regular eating patterns develop, weight tends to stabilize or drop due to newly consistent patterns of mindful eating. Don't fall for the myth that eating regularly or following a structured meal plan will cause weight gain. Structure a meal plan that includes three meals a day and two snacks with no more than three-hour gaps between meals. Make it feasible, realistic, and easy for your schedule. Incorporate as many "mindful meals" as possible into your daily life.

Skill Builder: Mindful Meal Planning

- Eat a minimum of three times a day. Eat breakfast and have small snacks. This is as important as putting gas in your car. Without fuel, your car isn't going to move, and neither will you. If you feel the urge to put something in your mouth, and you really aren't hungry, drink cold water. Sip the water slowly. Drink sparkling mineral water to feel the bubbles tickling your tongue. Buy flavored or vitamin-enriched water.

- Eat something small every three hours in accordance with your hunger. This prevents the urge to binge.

- Vegetarians and vegans are good examples of people who are mindful about their food choices. They actively adapt their relationship to food in a consistent and ongoing basis. If you are a vegetarian, make sure you obtain a well- rounded, sufficient amount of protein, vitamins, and minerals. Pay attention to your body's cues, and the signals it may send requesting more protein, calcium, or other vitamins and minerals.

- If you are not a vegetarian but claim you are, be honest about why. Sometimes, people hide behind being a vegetarian as a way to safely and quietly reduce their calorie intake. Other people don't question their refusal of food as intensely. If others inquire why you chose to become a vegetarian or vegan, notice your feelings and internal reactions. Don't hide behind this lifestyle choice.

- If you rely on coffee, tea, or caffeinated drinks to get you through the day, this is important to bring to your awareness. Pay attention to your energy levels. Think about whether you are using caffeine as a food substitute. Make it a goal to get enough energy via your food.

- Although everyone needs vitamins, it is best to get your vitamins from the original food source. The food primes your body to use the vitamins in the best possible way. When you salivate in response to food, it's an indication that your brain knows what is coming, and it sends signals throughout your body. Your brain doesn't react in the same way to vitamin pills. Eating whole foods is more mindful than taking vitamins because your entire body is integrated in the experience.

- Plan your meals for the day. Think about what you would prepare for someone else to use as a guide.

- When you are really hungry, eat something hot. Hot foods are often more filling and stimulate more internal sensation than cold foods.

- Avoid finger foods or appetizers. It's easier to overeat or binge on these foods because they skew your perception of the portion size.

- If you have trouble with binges, don't buy foods that are likely to make you binge or overeat, at least at first. Make your home and work space totally free of your favorite binge foods. Once you become more mindful and in better control of your eating, the presence of tempting foods shouldn't be a problem. However, at the beginning, make it as easy for yourself as is possible. If you have the urge to binge, and the food is present, *leave the room* for at least ten to twenty minutes. Get out of the environment.

- Consult a nutritionist to obtain information about the basic food groups (protein, dairy, fruits and vegetables, grains). This will help you understand what would be a "healthy" food plan for you. Get accurate information. Don't rely on what you read in trendy magazines.

- Avoid drugs and alcohol. These increase your vulnerability to eating mindlessly. Alcohol provides an abundance of mindless calories, and it reduces your ability to describe and observe your body sensations. Both alcohol and drugs alter and skew the precision, clarity, and purity of sensation that is necessary for mindful eating.

- Avoid caffeine. It is as much of a drug as alcohol. Too much caffeine can interfere with your perceptions and your ability to think clearly.

45
Stay on the Path and Keep Walking

"Fall down seven times, get up eight" is a Buddhist saying about resilience, persistence, and the ability to bounce back. If you read biographies about the lives of successful millionaires, their stories are remarkably similar. They all had a series of dramatic setbacks or "failures." For example, Milton Hershey, the founder of Hershey's chocolate, went bankrupt several times before making his fortune. The one quality that set such successful people apart from others, and contributed to their eventual success, was their ability to accept loss, feel the pain, learn from the experience, and jump right back up. In a similar way, mindful eating takes practice, and, in the beginning, you may not always succeed. However, if you keep trying to eat mindfully, you will succeed.

As Buddha said, "A jug fills drop by drop." In other words, mindful eating is a continual journey that requires an enormous amount of persistence. Potentially, healing your eating habits could be a lifelong activity. Also, be aware that regardless of how well you master mindfulness, it will be impossible to escape an unintentional bout of mindless eating, or the occasional lapse into old undereating habits. The doughnuts at work, the pizza ordered in, or a food that induces guilt feelings will temporarily tempt you back into a nonaware, self-indulgent mindset. When you realize what you have done, don't fall for the "Oh well, I've completely ruined it anyway" attitude.

Expect the occasional "out of the blue" mindless eating test, and consider it a challenge. It will happen. If problematic moments didn't occur, this would actually be a bad sign. Sometimes, you need to eat mindlessly to reestablish contact with mindful eating. Mindless eating will remind you of the benefits of controlled, aware eating. Think of the mindless eating as stepping into a pothole in the road. Tell yourself to keep walking. Think about it as if you were stepping out for a walk with a general, not specific, destination in mind. As the Buddha said, "If we are facing in the right direction, all we have to do is keep on walking."

Skill Builder: Let Accidental Mindless Eating Go

If you "slip up," be kind to yourself and let go of it. Don't focus on the past, regret, or guilt. Most importantly, don't try to push the mindless eating incident away. This is nonsense and goes directly in the face of mindfulness. You slipped up. It happened. Accept it and let go of it. You can use the experience to mindfully examine each sensation and to start again from this moment forward. You may have several, even many, slips on your path to mindful eating. Just pick yourself up whenever it happens, and keep on walking.

46
Hearing Your Inner Food Critic

Mindless eating can start off a stream of judgmental, malicious inner speech. Such "evaluative" thoughts about what you may have eaten are like a sportscaster's comments during the final seconds of a game. Instead of observing just what is happening sportscasters routinely describe mistakes in a disparaging, judgmental manner. In retrospect, they announce how the "right" play "should" have been executed. Similarly, your "inner food critic" may give you a play-by-play commentary about what you "should" or "should not" be eating. The critic can destroy your experience and enjoyment of eating.

"I can't believe I ate that, I'm such a fat, horrible person" is but one example of the harsh way that people can talk to themselves about their behavior. Turn your attention inward and take notice of what you say and think to yourself. When you begin to truly listen to yourself, you'll hear how often you make harsh, judgmental, false statements. Evaluation may trigger injurious, self-hating thoughts like, "I am such a horrible person for bingeing on junk food." Or, "Because I purged my food again, that proves what a weak-willed person I am." These judgmental remarks are damaging for many reasons, but mainly because thinking such thoughts pulls your senses away from fully experiencing eating. Thoughts like these are particularly dangerous when you allow them to whisper and repeat themselves subconsciously. Be aware and learn how subtle thoughts can have an impact on you.

Often, people mistakenly believe hypercritical judgments help control and limit mindless eating. There is a strong reluctance to put the inner food critic out of a job for fear that self-criticism is the only thing maintaining control. The inner food critic is a master at inducing little more than shame, self-hate, guilt, and regret. Ironically, these feelings are the prime instigators rather than stoppers of mindless eating.

Skill Builder: Silencing the Inner Food Critic with Compassion

Practice speaking to yourself in an sympathetic, uplifting manner. Gentle, positive inner speech is essential for any kind of mindful behavior, including eating. Be compassionate with yourself. Negative verbal commentary inhibits your ability to taste, smell, and enjoy your food in the moment. When you focus more on your critical thoughts than on the experience of eating, you are eating mindlessly. Truly listen to what you tell yourself, and examine how it influences what you eat. Buddha said, "Praise and blame, gain and loss, pleasure and sorrow come and go like the wind. To be happy, rest like a giant tree, in the midst of them all."

Sit still and turn your mind inward. Center yourself. Think about a recent difficult encounter with food. When your inner food critic speaks, what does it say? Is it yelling, whispering, nudging, urging, or sarcastic? Allow the thoughts to arise and just take note of them. Don't judge yourself for the thoughts but simply acknowledge the content and tone of your speech to yourself. Be mindful of the negative bodily and emotional impact of the words. Think about the way toxic, harsh inner speech distracts from your ability to taste and enjoy the food that sustains you.

Who Can Help You to Eat Mindfully?

Mastering mindful eating is no easy task. The more difficult it is for you to change your eating patterns and your mindset, the more likely it is that you would benefit from professional assistance. Although friends and family can be extremely helpful, sometimes talking to them about weight issues is tricky. When you talk about your own weight concerns and fears, it is often difficult for friends or family members to be sufficiently detached from their own weight fears and anxieties to really listen to what you say.

If you are unable to change your eating habits independently, or if meditating on the issues underlying your problem eating brings up overwhelming emotional reactions, it is important to seek professional help. A professional can assess what other factors need to be addressed. Professional help can be had from psychologists, psychiatrists, physicians, nurses, and nutritionists. A team of professionals is highly recommended. Each professional brings specialized training to an aspect of the mind, body, thoughts, or feelings, which woven together creates a holistic treatment. A medical professional is particularly valuable because antidepressants or other medications are necessary for some individuals. Lots of options exist including in-patient treatment for those who need to dedicate all of their attention at that moment.

Fluctuation in caloric intake is difficult on your mind and body. It can severely interfere with your concentration. A professional can tell you how to regain your focus. It is critical to seek additional help if you have mood issues or alcohol and/or drug problems. It is also critical if you are feeling suicidal, have had a dramatic loss of weight, are experiencing physical symptoms, or acting impulsively. These symptoms are likely to severely inhibit mindful eating because of the competing emotional demands.

Essentially, counseling is a way to break through your "stuck" thinking patterns. It helps you to articulate your feelings about food, and to identify patterns and connect the dots between the significant events in your life. As a counselor, I have guided many people through overcoming a wide range of eating issues. I feel honored by their trust and that they allowed me to help them combat this difficult problem.

When I think about my own role as a counselor, I imagine myself as a skydiving instructor. I am attached to the sky diver's back with an extra parachute just in case hers doesn't open. I allow the person to decide when she is going to jump, and how quickly she wants to open her own chute. I won't let her hit the ground, but I encourage all my clients to be mindfully in control. You may be afraid, and that's okay. I am sharing this image with you to let you know that professionals like me are here to help, not to judge, evaluate, or take away your control.

Mindful Eating:
Emergency Help

Providing specific instructions on what to do "in difficult moments" was an extremely important part of this book for me to write. Typically, my clients gain extraordinary insight into the origins and meaning of their food issues when they begin to practice mindful eating. However, they repeatedly have the same complaint, "What specifically can I do when I'm really struggling?" The following scenarios should walk you through some helpful steps. Refer back to the four parts of the book for expanded descriptions of each skill.

Scenario 1
Mindless Overeating Help

You have been sitting alone in front of your desk for several hours working on a project. You begin to think about the stash of chocolate candy hidden in the bottom of your desk drawer. Instantly, you forget what you are working on, and you can think about nothing but chocolate. In the past, opening up the desk drawer has led to you to uncontrolled, mindless eating.

Helping Steps

1. **Mindfully Meditate:** Begin to meditate in-the-moment. Stop everything you are doing (put down your pen, disconnect the phone) and devote your full attention to this issue.

2. **Breathing and Eating:** Slow down and do a quick breathing exercise. Focus and become aware of your body and your surroundings. Ask yourself what your breathing tells you about how you are feeling. Bring your attention to your breathing to recenter yourself and to increase your awareness.

3. **Mindful Hunger:** Ask yourself, "Am I really hungry?" Be mindful of the physical and logical cues that help you decide whether you are or not. When was the last time you ate? What is your body telling you? If the answer is, "No, I am not hungry," meditate on your feelings. Are you feeling bored by work or anxious about the project you are working on? What is going on? What else can you do to deal with what you're feeling? Will getting up from your desk and taking a short walk help? Is your body cramped from sitting still so long? Do you need to do some stretching?

4. **Mindful Cravings:** If the answer is, "Yes, I am hungry," think about your options. Identify what you really want to eat, and how much of it you need to satisfy your hunger.

5. **Mindful Awareness:** Tune into all of your senses as you eat, be in touch with the process of eating and with your body's reactions to the food.

6. **Mindful Activity:** Meditate on what is going on around you. What might "fill you up" just as well as food? If you are bored, do you need a break, would it help to call a friend, or to talk to a coworker for a few minutes? Make a plan.

7. **Mindful Imagery:** You know that starting to eat chocolate has led to treacherous binges in the past. Therefore, imagine a large, yellow and black DANGER road sign blocking the handle of your desk drawer. Meditate on that image.

Scenario 2
Mindless Undereating Help

You've been trying to lose weight and therefore skipped breakfast this morning. Your stomach is rumbling, and your head is beginning to throb. Although you would like to eat something, many thoughts stream through your mind like, "You're too fat to eat." You struggle between listening to your stomach and the judgmental voice inside your head.

Helping Steps

1. **Mindfulness of Your Body:** If your stomach is grumbling, think of this as a huge, red neon sign flashing, "I need food." When your stomach makes noise, that means you've waited too long. This puts you at greater risk of mindless eating. Stop what you are doing and focus completely on the physical cues your body is sending you. Be aware and observe. Take note of the sensations that you are feeling for next time. They will let you know you are really hungry. Breathe.

2. **Mindful Meditation:** Prevent yourself from going overboard. Carefully make a plan by thinking about what would be good for your body and what you need at this moment. Connect with your body. Spend time being inside your body and understanding what it needs. Watch your thoughts as outlined in Skill # 16.

3. **Mindful Speech:** Listen to the comments going through your mind. Notice your thoughts and feelings as you become aware of them. When they occur, label them for what they are, as "just a thought" or "just a feeling." If you are launching a personal attack on yourself, stop and instead think about the physical and emotional consequences of your actions. Transform your judgmental language into calm, soothing words. Talk yourself through it.

4. **Be Compassionate:** Speak kindly to yourself. Consider what you would tell someone else. If you have difficulty being sympathetic to yourself, call someone who will be. Avoiding criticism will help you to examine the situation with an open, mindful stance.

5. **Mindfulness of Emotions:** Examine the larger context of what is going on in this moment. Clearly, you are hungry, but what else is going on internally? Think about what happened in the events surrounding this moment. Do what is called "walking backward and forward," as discussed in Skill # 27. Think first about the present moment, and then think deeply about your feelings in the preceding moments. What prompted this struggle?

6. **Acceptance of Self:** Eating can induce many negative feelings about yourself and your body. In this moment, acknowledge that at some level you simply must accept

your body as it is. You are in control of making that choice. You don't have to love every aspect of your body to respect it and treat it well. Think about how the food is going to benefit how well your body functions. Your headache will stop. Use imagery to imagine where the food will travel once it is inside.

Scenario 3
Mindless Chaotic Eating Help

A group of friends get together one night at your home to watch a video and eat a pizza. They order your favorite pizza toppings. Everyone is eating several slices, which leads you to eat two more pieces than you typically would have eaten. After they leave, you eat another slice, despite not being hungry. You begin to feel the urge to rid yourself of the heavy pizza and the too-full feeling.

Helpful Steps

1. **Mindful Eating Journey:** When you lapse back into mindless eating, it may feel as if you are beginning your journey all over again or, even worse, that you have completely strayed off the path. This is not true. Once you've learned about mindfulness you won't forget it. It's a matter of reapplying principles. At this point, you need to forgive yourself. Most people advocate for "forgive and forget." Mindfulness doesn't do that. Instead, it urges you to "forgive and accept." Don't try to push away your feelings. Accept all that you are feeling.

2. **Mindfulness of Your Body:** Feeling too full is a common reason people get the urge to eliminate their food. A much healthier way to deal with the uncomfortable feelings is to meditate. Stop and meditate on the emotional components of your bodily feelings. Getting in touch with your feelings will be useful for preventing overeating next time.

3. **Mindfulness of Feelings:** The urge to purge the food is a quick way of dealing with the anxiety that is aroused by eating unnecessary calories. It is important to be mindful and to meditate on the entire evening. What feelings prompted you to eat mindlessly, particularly after your friends left? What tends to trigger eating when you aren't even hungry? Is this a pattern?

4. **Mindfulness of Physical Consequences:** Purging is instigated by the negative emotions that arise when you realize you ate mindlessly. Purging is a dangerous, mindless activity. When individuals first begin purging, they are more aware of their negative feelings and their body's physical reactions. Over time, the individual disconnects from the moment-to-moment discomfort of purging, and anticipates feeling better, soothed, or relieved that the extra calories are gone. Acknowledge what purging does to your body in a nonjudgmental way. Advocate for your health.

5. **Mindful Activity:** The urge to feel better quickly by purging the food is tempting and sometimes feels difficult to control. Therefore, it is important to refocus your mind on other things. Get out of the house. Take a walk, listen to music, or visit someone. Find a soothing activity to engage in that will help you reduce your anxiety about the entire experience.

Scenario 4
Stepping Back in The
Midst of Temptation

Imagine you are in the kitchen and you are wrestling with the temptation to reach for a bag of cookies sitting on the shelf. You think, "I just want one taste." Here is a technique to help you take a "step back" and walk you through some decisions. This is a good tactic to help you examine any difficult eating dilemma.

Helpful Steps

1. **Mindfully Step Back:** Imagine yourself actively taking a step back from the situation. Why is stepping back important? When stressed or overwhelmed, people tend to revert to "autopilot." This means eating or behaving in their habitual way. Essentially, you "react" automatically, rather than investigating all the pertinent and critical information. Stepping back helps you to obtain, thoughtfully and consciously, all the information you need to identify an array of solutions. Stepping back is carefully responding with diligent thought, rather than robotically reacting. Identify how you would "typically react."

2. **Mindful Speech:** Describe aloud what is happening to you both internally and externally. Use detail, description, and lots of adjectives. Rely on your senses: sight, smell, sound, taste, and touch. Use vivid details, as if you were describing the scene to someone with his eyes closed. Example: "I really want a cookie. I'm in the kitchen standing in front of the cabinet. I am afraid I am going to overeat and finish all the cookies

in the box. I feel nervous, and my hands are shaking. I'm sweating with anxiety, and I'm pacing around because I don't know what to do."

3. **Mindful Acceptance:** The "sixth" and most important sensory organ is your mind. Describe what you are feeling and thinking. Think about the situation objectively without inserting any judgmental statements. Don't distort the description with statements that what is happening is "bad" or "wrong." Be compassionate with yourself. Example: "I feel really hungry, and I am frustrated. This is a really tough situation for me. In the past, I know this kind of situation has ended up with me feeling really bad. It's okay to feel this way."

4. **Mindful Thoughts:** Describe clearly what you want. Verbalizing is like translating a foreign text into your own language. Read the situation, pause, describe it using your own words. Example: "I want to eat a cookie but I don't want to binge or overeat. How do I feel? This really stinks!"

5. **Mindful Planning:** Describe your options. Consider every scenario. *Example:* "I could binge, leave the room, eat something else, have one cookie and stop, call someone, watch TV, or go for a walk."

6. **Mindful Choosing:** Describe your choice. Make a decision. Visualize that decision. Imagine carrying out your decision. *Example:* "I will eat just one, and leave the kitchen to prevent myself from eating too many." Close your eyes and picture yourself walking out of the room.

7. **Letting Go:** Describe what you need to release. *Example:* "I may not feel completely satisfied in the moment, but I will feel better about myself after the urge subsides."

Resources

Eating and Mindfulness

Visit my website at www.eatingmindfully.com

General eating issues information can be found at the following sites:

www.mirror-mirror.org

www.aedweb.org

www.anred.com

www.nationaleatingdisorders.org

www.edreferral.com

Referrals

1-800-THERAPIST
www.1-800-therapist.com

Please note that clinical examples are fictitious or have been altered to conceal the identity of the individual.

References

Alexander, W. 1997. *Cool Water: Alcoholism, Mindfulness and Ordinary Recovery*. Boston: Shambhala Publications, Inc.

Bourne, E. 1995. *The Anxiety and Phobia Workbook*. Second edition. Oakland, Calif.: New Harbinger Publishing.

Burns, D. 1999. Preface by Aaron Beck. *Feeling Good: The New Mood Therapy*. New York: Avon Books.

Carlat, D. J., and C. A. Carmargo. 1991. Review of bulimia nervosa in males. *American Journal of Psychiatry* 148:831–843.

Costin, C. 1999. *The Eating Disorder Sourcebook: A Comprehensive Guide to the Causes, Treatments and Prevention of Eating Disorders*. Second edition. Los Angeles: Lowell House.

Crow, S., B. Praus, and P. Thuras. 1999. Mortality from eating disorders: A 5 to 10 year record linkage study. *International Journal of Eating Disorders* 26:97–101.

Gunarantana, B. 2001. *Eight Mindful Steps to Happiness*. Boston: Wisdom Publications.

Hayes, S., K. Wilson, and K. Strosahl. 1999. *Acceptance and Commitment Therapy: An Experiential Approach to Behavior Change*. New York: Guilford Press.

Hendrix, H. 2001. *Getting the Love You Want: A Guide for Couples*. New York: Henry Holt & Company.

Kabat-Zinn, J. 1990. *Full Catastrophe Living: Using the Wisdom of Your Body and Mind to Face Stress, Pain and Illness*. New York: Dell Publishing.

Linehan, M. 1993. *Cognitive-Behavioral Treatment for Borderline Personality Disorder*. New York: Guilford Press.

Marcus, M., and E. McCabe. 2002. Dialectical Behavioral Therapy (DBT) in the Treatment of Eating Disorders. Paper presented at the International Conference of Eating Disorders and Clinical Teaching Days. Boston: April 25 2002.

Sandbeck, T. 1993. *The Deadly Diet: Recovering from Anorexia and Bulimia*. Oakland, Calif.: New Harbinger Publications.

Smolak, L., M. Levine, and R. Strigel-Moore. 1996. *The Developmental Psychopathology of Eating Disorders: Implications for Research, Prevention and Treatment*. Hillsdale, NJ.: England Lawrence Earlbaum Associates.

Thich Nhat Hanh. 1990. *Present Moment Wonderful Moment: Mindfulness for Daily Life*. Berkeley, Calif.: Parallax Press.

Wiser, S., and C. Telch. 1999. Dialectical behavioral therapy for binge-eating disorder. *Journal of Clinical Psychology* 55: 755–768.

Wolpe, J. 1958. *Psychotherapy by Reciprocal Inhibition*. Stanford, Calif.: Stanford University Press.

Zerbe, K. 1995. *The Body Betrayed: A Deeper Understanding of Women, Eating Disorders and Treatment*. Carlsbad, Calif.: Gurze Books.

Zindel, V., M. Segal, G. Williams, and J. Teasdale. 2001. *Mindfulness-Based Cognitive Therapy for Depression*. New York: Guilford Press.

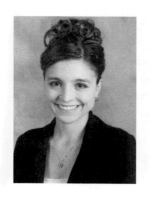

Susan Albers, Psy.D., a University of Denver graduate, has specialized in eating disorder treatment at the University of Notre Dame, Ohio Wesleyan University, and Stanford University Counseling and Psychological Services. Albers maintains a private practice where she treats men and women with Eating-related issues and mood disorders.

Some Other New Harbinger Titles

The Cyclothymia Workbook, Item 383X, $18.95

The Matrix Repatterning Program for Pain Relief, Item 3910, $18.95

Transforming Stress, Item 397X, $10.95

Eating Mindfully, Item 3503, $13.95

Living with RSDS, Item 3554 $16.95

The Ten Hidden Barriers to Weight Loss, Item 3244 $11.95

The Sjogren's Syndrome Survival Guide, Item 3562 $15.95

Stop Feeling Tired, Item 3139 $14.95

Responsible Drinking, Item 2949 $18.95

The Mitral Valve Prolapse/Dysautonomia Survival Guide,
Item 3031 $14.95

Stop Worrying Abour Your Health, Item 285X $14.95

The Vulvodynia Survival Guide, Item 2914 $15.95

The Multifidus Back Pain Solution, Item 2787 $12.95

Move Your Body, Tone Your Mood, Item 2752 $17.95

The Chronic Illness Workbook, Item 2647 $16.95

Coping with Crohn's Disease, Item 2655 $15.95

The Woman's Book of Sleep, Item 2493 $14.95

The Trigger Point Therapy Workbook, Item 2507 $19.95

Fibromyalgia and Chronic Myofascial Pain Syndrome, second edition,
Item 2388 $19.95

Kill the Craving, Item 237X $18.95

Call **toll free, 1-800-748-6273,** or log on to our online bookstore
at **www.newharbinger.com** to order. Have your Visa or Mastercard
number ready. Or send a check for the titles you want to New
Harbinger Publications, Inc., 5674 Shattuck Ave., Oakland, CA 94609
Include $4.50 for the first book and 75¢ for each additional book, to
cover shipping and handling. (California residents please include
appropriate sales tax.) Allow two to five weeks for delivery.

Prices subject to change without notice.